EATING for EYE HEALTH

The Macular Degeneration Cookbook

EATING for EYE HEALTH

The Macular Degeneration Cookbook

Ita Buttrose & Vanessa Jones

Published in 2014.
First published in Australia in 2009 by
New Holland Publishers (Australia) Pty Ltd
London • Sydney • Auckland

www.newhollandpublishers.com

131-151 Great Titchfield Street London WIW 5BB United Kingdom
1/66 Gibbes Street Chatswood NSW 2067 Australia
5/39 Woodside Ave Northcote Auckland 0627 New Zealand

National Library of Australia Cataloguing-in-Publication Data: Author: Buttrose, Ita and Jones, Vanessa.

ISBN: 9781742575209

Title: Eating for Eye Health / Ita Buttrose and Vanessa Jones. ISBN: 9781742575209 (pbk.)
Subjects:Cookery.
Retinal degeneration--Diet therapy.
Retinal degeneration--Nutritional aspects. Dewey Number: 641.5632

Publisher: Fiona Schultz
Editor: Kay Proos
Junior editor: Ashlea Wallington
Designer: Lorena Susak
Photography: New Holland Image Library/Graeme Gillies Cooking and Styling: Vanessa Jones and Sue Forster-Wright
Production manager: Olga Dementiev
Printer: Toppan Leefung Printing Limited

10 9 8 7 6 5 4 3

Photographs on pages 9, 32, 36, 42, 52, 88, 90, 96, 97, 124, 144, 158 and 168 by Tony Sheffield. Reprinted by courtesy of Highlife Magazine, Bowral, NSW, Australia

New Holland Publishers would like to acknowledge the generosity of Villeroy & Boch, Genevieve Lethu, www.genevievelethu.com, Claudio's Seafoods at Sydney Fish Markets, Lane Cove West Fruit Market.

Follow New Holland Publishers on
Facebook: www.facebook.com/NewHollandPublishers

In memory of my father, Charles Buttrose, who suffered from macular degeneration. I wish I knew then what I know now about the best way to go about preventing this disease.

Ita Buttrose

For Nona, my English grandmother.

Vanessa Jones

ACKNOWLEDGEMENTS

No book ever just happens. Many people help contribute to making what seems like a good idea become reality. The authors particularly want to thank Dr Paul Beaumont who has provided invaluable guidance on diet and nutrition. As a founding Director of the Macular Disease Foundation Australia his passion for treating and supporting people with the disease is legendary and his enthusiasm for this book has been terrific. Our thanks to providores Matt Brown's Greens and Craig Cummins Seafood for supplying Vanessa's first class produce and Lisa Yates, the dietitian at Nuts For Life for her advice and expertise on nuts and nutrition. Thanks also to David Smith, the Managing Director of Canongate Partners Pty Ltd for giving us access to photographs from Highlife magazine and a very big thank you to the staff and members of the Union, University & Schools Club of Sydney. The kitchen staff has helped Vanessa test many of the recipes and the club's members have been willing and constructive tasters and consequently have helped with the compilation of the recipes in this book. Finally our sincere thanks to those people living with macular degeneration who have been our inspiration for this book.

FOREWORD

Since becoming patron of the Macular Disease Foundation Australia in 2005 I have become aware of how widespread the disease is and how much ignorance about it exists in our community.

It's odd really because so many people suffer from it—millions in fact—yet many people simply take their eye health for granted. I have made it my mission to tell people about macular degeneration and encourage them to have regular eye checks and adopt an eye friendly diet and lifestyle.

My father was in his mid-eighties when he lost his central vision to macular degeneration. It changed his life. As a journalist and author he had always started his day reading a couple of newspapers. Suddenly this was no longer possible.

As a journalist and author myself I couldn't imagine not being able to ever read again. I was as devastated about Dad's fate as he was.

One of Dad's sisters also had macular degeneration and, a few years ago, their youngest brother was also diagnosed. Fortunately the sight of one of my uncle's eyes has been saved with the help of a treatment now available for wet macular degeneration. This has been a major breakthrough in the management of the disease and my uncle's doctor has been able to stabilise his vision. If only this treatment had been around to help Dad, how happier the last years of his life would have been.

One thing I have noticed is how few people know that a family history of the disease brings with it a high risk. When I tell them that I have a 50 per cent chance of getting it too, most people are usually shocked. My children are equally at risk and consequently we all do some kind of regular exercise, watch our weight and follow the eating program recommended by the Foundation.

This is not a deprivation method of eating; you won't feel hungry. There are some wonderful recipes for cooking and serving vegetables, fruit and fish in this book and once you get the hang of eating this way you will discover how delicious and satisfying it is. It's wise to maintain a healthy weight. I usually exercise every day—I might walk for an hour on some days and swim several laps on another. I also work out at my local gym a couple of times a week. You don't have to follow my regime though—work out your own but at the very least, do try to walk for at least 30 minutes three times a week. If you get into the habit of exercising regularly you will feel much better for it.

I get my macula checked annually and when my ophthalmic surgeon tells me my 'macula is in pristine condition' his words are music to my ears and I just about dance out of his surgery one of the happiest women in the world!

As the Foundation's patron I am excited about the opportunity that *Eating for Eye Health* gives us to help raise awareness of macular degeneration. I have enjoyed collaborating with Vanessa Jones—one of Australia's up-and coming young chefs for whom I predict a brilliant future—in making this project a reality.

We are both proud of this book and all that it offers to people who want the very best for their eye health.

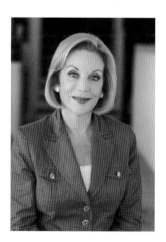

Ita Buttrose AO, OBE
Australian of the Year 2013

FOREWORD

When I was asked to produce this cookbook for the Macular Disease Foundation Australia it was a dream come true. Ever since I was 14, when I bought my first copy of *Vogue Entertaining* and discovered the inspiring world of food, my long-term ambition has been to write cookbooks and to become a food stylist.

Luck has played an important role in my career. When I was a sous chef at Milton Park Country House Hotel, Bowral, in the Southern Highlands of New South Wales, I prepared and styled the hotel's advertisements for the regional magazine, *Highlife*, with the help of the magazine's chief photographer, Tony Sheffield.

This led to me meeting Ita Buttrose, then the Editor of *Highlife*, who asked me to become the magazine's food writer and stylist. What an opportunity! Writing about food is something that gives me enormous joy.

It's through my connection with Ita that this cookbook has come to life. As Patron of the Macular Disease Foundation Australia she recommended me for the job. Ita has been a great mentor and I want to thank her for her faith in me and for all her hard work, advice and editing of *Eating for Eye Health*. She has been amazing to work with.

Good eye health is something I'm passionate about because my uncle, Laurie James, has macular degeneration and I'm well aware of its devastating effects. Macular degeneration has stopped Uncle Laurie from doing many basic daily tasks, including driving, which has been an enormous blow to him. I've promised him the first copy of this book when it's published.

I've concentrated on the preferred ingredients for eye health in my recipes and you'll find that many include salmon, which is rich in omega-3 fatty acids and also lutein-rich spinach. Both omega-3 fatty acids and lutein are important for good eye health. Always use a good quality extra virgin olive oil. I like to use Australian products which are some of the best in the world. Wherever possible I've also used ingredients that represent a healthier choice.

I like to use salt when I cook but the choice is yours. My recipes work without it. I also like to use picked rather than chopped leaves of soft herbs like parsley and rocket in many of my dishes because whole leaves give a better texture and flavour.

I love being a chef. My world revolves around food—its incredible smells, tastes and flavours—and memorable dining experiences. Working in a kitchen brigade has been compared to sailing in a ship full of pirates. I couldn't agree more and there's nothing better than being the captain!

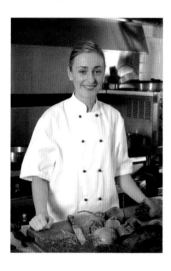

Vanessa Jones

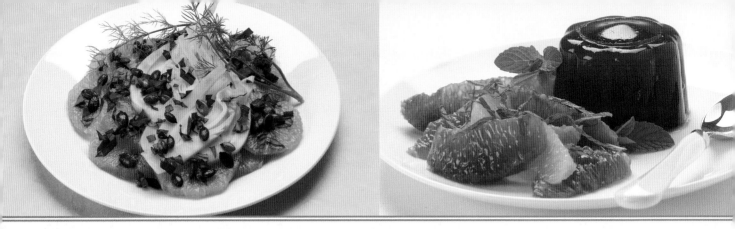

CONTENTS

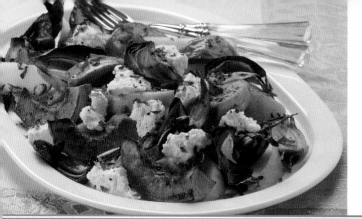
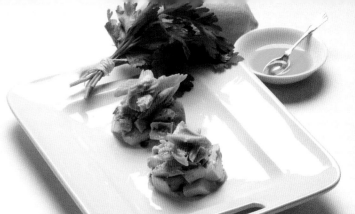

INTRODUCTION

WHAT WE KNOW ABOUT MACULAR DEGENERATION

Macular degeneration is the leading cause of blindness and severe vision loss in developed countries. Over one million Australians, or one in seven people over 50, show some evidence of macular degeneration.

In addition to age, the risk factors for macular degeneration are genetics and smoking. If you have a direct family history there is a 50 per cent chance of developing the disease, and smokers are three to four times more likely to develop macular degeneration.

Macular degeneration affects the macula which is the central part of the retina—the light-sensitive tissue at the back of the eye which processes all visual images. The macula is responsible for our ability to read, recognise faces, drive and see colours clearly. You are reading this cookbook using your macula. Macular degeneration causes progressive damage resulting in loss of central vision. Peripheral vision is not affected.

There are two forms of macular degeneration—'dry' and 'wet'. Dry macular degeneration results in a gradual loss of central vision. Wet macular degeneration is characterised by a sudden loss of vision and is caused by abnormal blood vessels growing into the retina.

In recent times, breakthrough drug treatments have changed the landscape of wet macular degeneration. This has brought amazing benefits but more research is needed in order to move closer to developing a cure for this disease.

We do know however that a few simple changes to lifestyle and diet can help people suffering from both forms of macular degeneration and also people at risk of getting the disease. Don't smoke, avoid being overweight, do some exercise on a regular basis, eat a healthy, well-balanced diet, limit your intake of fats, eat fish two to three times a week, dark green leafy vegetables and fresh fruit daily plus a handful of nuts weekly. Protect yourself from the sun and wear sunglasses.

These easy to put into place measures are all good for your overall health, your eye health and particularly your macula.

Evidence now exists to support the use of lutein, zeaxanthin (carotenoids), selenium and omega–3 fatty acids to improve the health of the macula and thus reduce the risk of developing macular degeneration. In spite of their fancy names you'll find them in everyday food items. Lutein and zeaxanthin are in dark leafy greens such as kale, spinach and silverbeet as well as sweet corn and egg yolks. Selenium is found in nuts—especially Brazil nuts—and omega–3 fatty acids are found in fish.

With the help of the culinary talents of Vanessa Jones, this book will show you how enjoyable it can be to eat healthy meals that will help to reduce your risk of losing your vision.

Dr Paul Beaumont, AM
Ophthalmologist

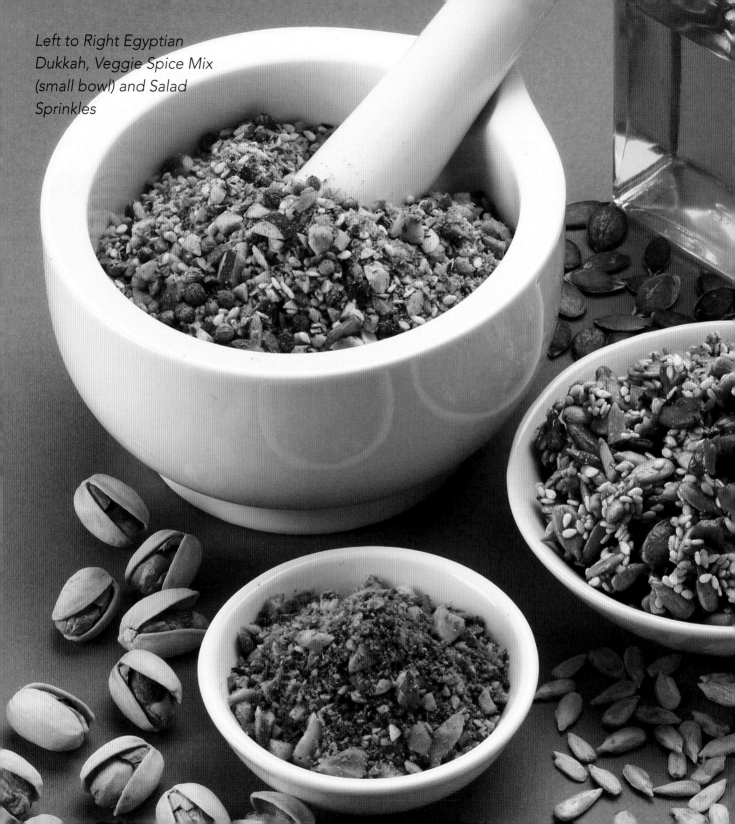

Left to Right Egyptian Dukkah, Veggie Spice Mix (small bowl) and Salad Sprinkles

One

GETTING DOWN TO BASICS

When I was learning my trade I was told that a smart cook's secret weapon is a well-stocked pantry. Over the years I've found this to be true. Every pantry should have basic ingredients like flour, rice, pasta, couscous, herbs, and oils and if you add some salad sprinkles or an exotic spice mix that you have made yourself to your pantry stock, you'll always be able to turn a simple meal into something quite impressive with a minimum of fuss.

A well-stocked pantry means you'll never be caught out when guests turn up unexpectedly. I often tell my friends to drop in whenever they feel like it and some do on a regular basis because they love my fish cakes. Fortunately these are easily whipped up with a tin of salmon, a must-have item in my pantry. I always have a few tins of tomatoes, chickpeas, lentils, mushrooms and asparagus on hand too, so I won't be caught short. (See Chapter Six, Meals in a Hurry.)

Olive oil is an essential item in my pantry because I use it in so many of my recipes. I love trying different brands from different regions with their varied and complex flavours reflecting the area where the olives are grown. Just like wine, olive oil is a product of its surrounds and is affected by soil and climate.

Good quality extra virgin olive oil comes from the first pressing of the finest olives and is best used as 'finishing oil'. It is wonderful for dressing salad leaves, drizzling over fresh pasta or simply using as a dip for crusty bread. It never should be heated and used only with dishes that are ready for eating.

Use light olive oil for marinating, frying and baking. It has a more subtle flavour and won't overpower the food.

All olive oil should be stored in airtight bottles in a dark, cool pantry. Kept in the right conditions olive oil can be stored for up to one year.

You should also include a variety of nuts and seeds in your pantry stock. When you use them for cooking they should be toasted to bring out their best flavour. The best way to do this is to place them in a dry frying pan on medium to low heat for two to three minutes or until lightly browned and fragrant.

After toasting, nuts and seeds lose their flavour if stored too long so use them fairly quickly. Keep stored in airtight containers in a dark, cool pantry.

Don't forget to also keep a few basic items in your freezer. Frozen spinach is useful because it can replace fresh spinach in most recipes. Other handy items are baby peas, pesto, pastry, corn, uncooked salmon fillets, frozen mixed berries, bird's-eye chilli and lemon grass.

HEALTHY EATING

Cooking with healthy ingredients should be part of day-to-day life. Healthy eating should accommodate personal preferences as well as any special dietary requirements*. So remember that you may like to:
- Substitute the butter or oils with a personal preference
- Reduce quantities of high fat ingredients such as blue cheese
- Omit added salt
- Choose low salt ingredients

But of course sometimes we all need a special treat so the occasional indulgence is perfectly fine.

*Always consult your doctor when making any significant changes to your diet or lifestyle.

SPICE AND ALL THINGS NICE

I couldn't imagine cooking without spices. They add such zing to a dish. There's nothing better than lightly poached peaches with fresh, fragrant cinnamon quills, or Brussels sprouts with a dash of butter and a sprinkle of nutmeg, or the exotic taste of a panna cotta infused with a little star anise.

I first discovered spices riding in a cycle rickshaw through a maze of Indian streets in Old Delhi, leading to Khari Baoli, Asia's largest wholesale spice market, where something like 88 per cent of the world's spices are traded.

I was captivated by the hustle and bustle of the place and the shopkeepers who sold an extraordinary array of spices, nuts, seeds and herbs. The colours and the smells were amazing. Nothing could hold me back from exploring what was on offer—masses of fresh vanilla bean, turmeric root, star anise, lotus seeds, nutmeg and the freshest cinnamon quills.

Just like spices, nuts and seeds enhance a dish and I use them a lot when I'm cooking. I often use pine nuts in my recipes because they just taste so good—their sweet buttery flavour is wonderful in just about anything. I like using sesame and pumpkin seeds too because they're extremely versatile and can be added to both sweet and savoury dishes.

If you're watching calories you can use spices as a substitute for butter and oil. They also can be used instead of salt in many recipes. Nuts and seeds make a tasty substitute for flour and breadcrumbs.

SALAD SPRINKLE MIX

Makes ½ cup

Sprinkle this over your favourite lettuce salad and drizzle with olive oil.

¼ cup sunflower seeds
2 tablespoons sesame seeds
2 tablespoons pumpkin seeds

2 tablespoons soy sauce
1 tablespoon honey
1 tablespoon olive oil

Pre-heat oven to moderately slow, 160°C (325°F) Gas Mark 3. Mix all the ingredients until well combined.
Line a flat tray with baking paper.
Spoon the ingredients on to the tray and cook for 12 minutes or until golden. Allow to cool. Use immediately or store in an airtight container.

VEGGIE SPICE MIX

Makes 1½ –2 cups

Toss this through steamed vegetables and then drizzle with olive oil or sprinkle it on vegetable soup for an extra kick. Veggie Spice Mix also makes an excellent substitute for salt and pepper.

200g (6½oz) Brazil nuts, crushed
1 tablespoon black mustard seeds
1 tablespoon cumin powder

1 tablespoon turmeric powder
1 tablespoon cayenne pepper
½ tablespoon sea salt

Pre-heat oven to moderately slow, 160°C (325°F) Gas Mark 3.
Line a flat tray with baking paper and put the nuts, spices and salt on the tray and cook for 7 minutes.
Allow to cool and store in an airtight container.

EGYPTIAN DUKKAH

Makes 1½ cups

Egyptian dukkah spice mix is available at specialty delicatessens; however this quick and easy recipe costs a fraction of the price. It also makes for interesting talk at the dinner table. Serve a bowl of Egyptian dukkah and olive oil with bread, preferably warm sourdough. The idea is to first dip the bread into the oil and then into the dukkah. Dukkah is best served with pre-dinner drinks.

100g (3½oz) Brazil nuts
50g (2oz) pistachio kernels
100g (3½oz) sesame seeds

50g (2oz) coriander (cilantro) seeds
50g (2oz) cumin powder
1 tablespoon sea salt

Pre-heat oven to moderately slow, 160°C (325°F) Gas Mark 3. Line a flat tray with baking paper.
Place the Brazil nuts and pistachio kernels on the tray and cook for 5 minutes.
Sprinkle the sesame and coriander seeds and cumin over the nuts and cook for a further 5 minutes.
Remove from the oven and allow to cool.
Using a mortar and pestle crush the spices and nuts to form a coarse powder. Add the salt and mix until combined. Store in an airtight container.

Note: Dukkah has a short shelf life so only make it in small quantities.

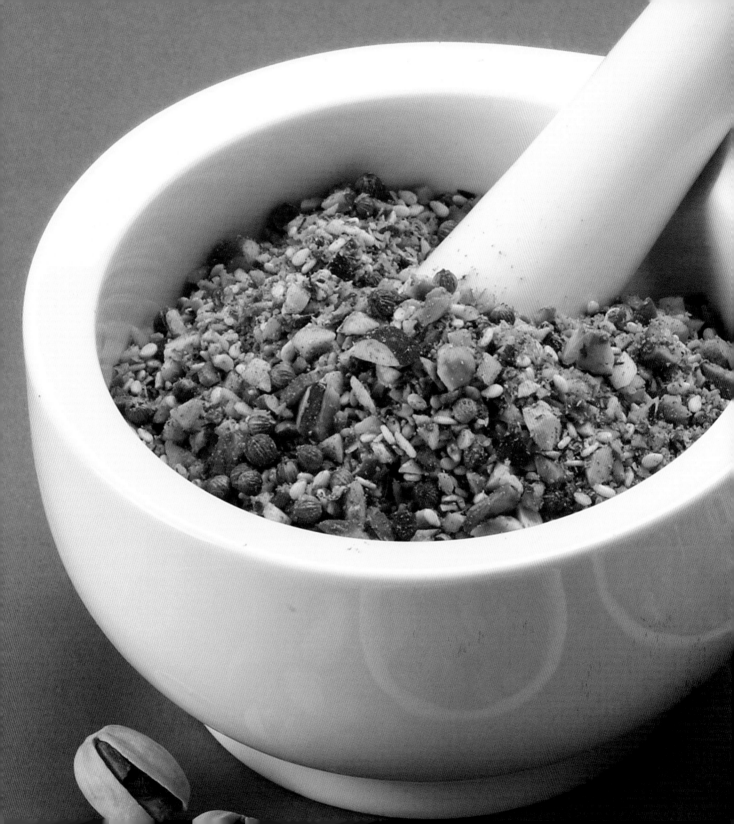

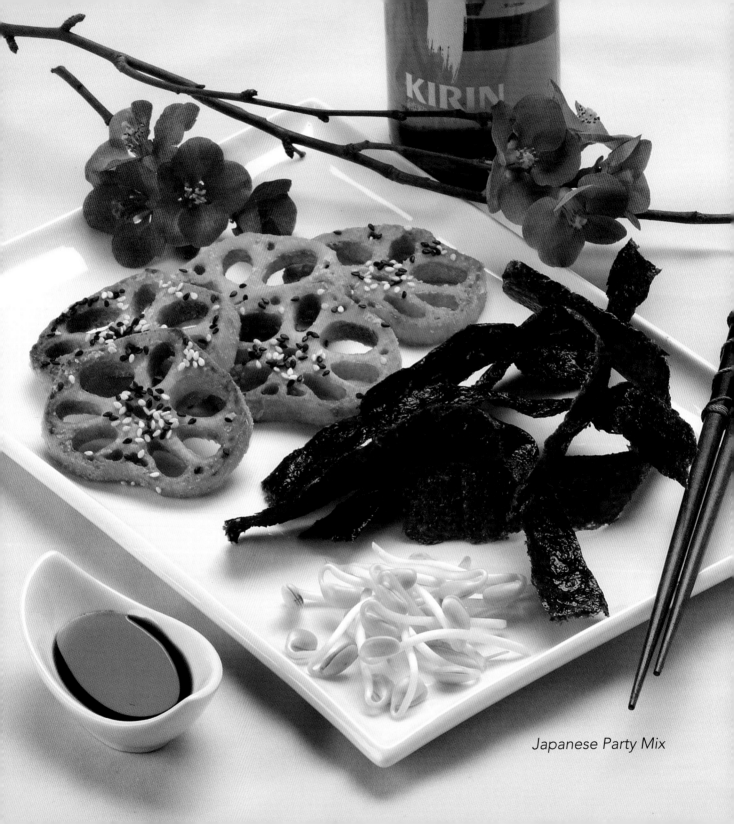

Japanese Party Mix

SNACK TIME

One of the best things about my snack suggestions is the sensational smell that fills the house when I'm preparing them. And they're good for you too—Brazil nuts are an excellent source of selenium, which is good for macular health. Like walnuts, pine nuts and almonds, Brazil nuts are also high in essential fatty acids which are beneficial for your eyes and almonds are an excellent source of vitamin E which is also essential for your eye health. Soybeans are not only low in calories but are also a source of iron, zinc and selenium.

I always serve snacks before dinner as they seem to stimulate people's hunger and get them ready for the main event! I choose nibbles that complement whatever dish I'm cooking. For instance, if I'm having a curry night I offer Bollywood Bites but if I'm doing a sushi menu I offer soybeans.

Snacks shouldn't fill you up. The trick is not to eat too much of them. Take your time to enjoy the flavour and taste the texture.

SPICY BRAZIL NUTS

Makes 3½ –4 cups

These are best served while still warm, however leftovers can be stored in an airtight container until needed.

    500g (1lb) Brazil nuts
    2 tablespoons light olive oil
    1 tablespoon poppy seeds
    2 tablespoons Egyptian dukkah (see note)

Pre-heat oven to moderate, 180°C (350°F) Gas Mark 4.
Put the nuts in a small bowl and coat with the olive oil, then place on an ungreased baking tray and sprinkle with poppy seeds and dukkah.
Cook for 8 minutes or until slightly browned and aromatic.

Note: See Spice and All Things Nice in this chapter for dukkah.

SPICED CHICKPEAS

These are best served straight from the oven.

300g (9½oz) tinned chickpeas
2 tablespoons Cajun spice powder
2 tablespoons light olive oil

Pre-heat oven to slow, 150°C (300°F) Gas Mark 2. Drain and wash the chickpeas in cold water.
Mix the spice powder and oil together and pour over the chickpeas until they are well coated. Place the chickpeas on an ungreased baking tray and cook for 20 minutes.

TRAIL MIX

¼ cup honey, warmed
¼ cup (60ml/2fl oz) light olive oil
200g (6½oz) Brazil nuts
100g (3½oz) raw almonds

100g (3½oz) dried apricots
100g (3½oz) dried figs, cut in halves
50g (2oz) shredded coconut

Pre-heat oven to moderate, 180°C (350°F) Gas Mark 4. Mix the honey and oil together in a small bowl.
Combine the nuts, dried fruit and coconut in a large bowl.
Add the honey and oil mix, lightly coating the nut and fruit mixture.
Spoon on to a baking tray that has been lined with baking paper, spread the mixture out evenly and cook for 10 minutes.
Allow to cool then store in an airtight container.

JAPANESE PARTY MIX

This is great served as a side dish with a bowl of miso soup or as a pre-dinner munchie.

100g (3½ oz) fresh lotus root (see note)
1 tablespoon wasabi powder
¼ cup plain flour
1 teaspoon sea salt
2 tablespoons light olive oil

2 sheets nori seaweed,
    cut into 2cm (¾in) strips
1 tablespoon white sesame seeds, toasted
1 tablespoon black sesame seeds,
    toasted
Soy sauce

Wash the dirt off the lotus root, peel and cut it into 1cm (½in) slices.
Combine the wasabi powder, flour and salt in a bowl then roll the lotus root slices in the flour mix until well coated.
Heat the olive oil in a shallow frying pan and cook the lotus root for 3 minutes or until golden brown. Cook the nori strips in the same oil for 30 seconds or until crisp. Place the lotus root and nori on absorbent paper to remove any excess oil. Sprinkle with the sesame seeds and serve with a small bowl of soy sauce for dipping.

Note: Lotus root is available fresh in Australia all through winter.

BOLLYWOOD BITES

Serve nuts spiced with Indian flavours and bring out your inner Bollywood fantasies!

200g (6½oz) peanuts
200g (6½oz) Brazil nuts
1 teaspoon turmeric powder
1 teaspoon cumin powder
1 teaspoon sea salt

1 teaspoon chilli powder
1 teaspoon garam masala powder
  (see note)
2 tablespoons light olive oil

Pre-heat oven to moderate, 180°C (350°F) Gas Mark 4.
Mix all the ingredients together in a large bowl until the nuts are evenly coated with the spices.
Place the mixture on an ungreased baking tray, spread out evenly and cook for 10 minutes or until golden brown.
Serve straight from the oven.

Note: Garam masala is a spice blend of cardamom, Indian bay leaves, black pepper, cumin, coriander and cinnamon. It is available at Asian grocers and most supermarkets.

SOYBEANS

I could eat these beans by the kilo! They are deliciously addictive and just the thing for tasty pre-dinner nibbles. I prefer soybeans served hot, however on a warm summer's day they are delicious if you pop them in the refrigerator for a couple of hours after cooking and serve them chilled. Just like green peas the outer shell of the soybean is discarded and only the beans are eaten so the ideal way to eat soybeans is to squeeze the pods and pop the beans straight into your mouth. They go perfectly with an icy-cold Japanese beer!

500g (1lb) soybeans (edamame pods), frozen

Sea salt

Bring a large saucepan of water to the boil, add the frozen beans and cook for 4–5 minutes.
Drain, and sprinkle the soybeans with a pinch of sea salt.

Note: Soybeans are best bought frozen from Asian grocers.

If You Have A Sweet Tooth...

NUT PRALINE

Makes 1–1½ cups

Praline can be eaten as a substitute for desserts. I like to crush praline and fold it through ice cream.

1 cup (250ml/8fl oz) water
1 cup caster sugar
100g (3½oz) almonds, roughly chopped
100g (3½oz) Brazil nuts, roughly chopped

Combine the water and sugar in a medium saucepan and boil for 10–15 minutes or until the sugar mixture has turned a light blonde colour.
Working very quickly, add the nuts, stirring all the time with a wooden spoon.
Put a sheet of baking paper on a heatproof bench (the draining side of the kitchen sink is ideal) and spoon the mixture on to it, then smooth it out with a wooden spoon.
Allow to cool then snap praline into smaller shards and keep in an airtight container.

Note: Praline can be stored in an airtight container for up to one week.

QUICK WAYS WITH CELERY

- Serve thinly sliced apple, fennel and celery on toasted rye bread.

- A glass of tomato juice with a little freshly ground black pepper and a celery stick makes a refreshing drink.

- Cut celery into bite-size pieces and fill with blue cheese topped with a sprinkle of Brazil nuts or ricotta mixed with grated carrot and flaked almonds and topped with a little freshly ground black pepper.

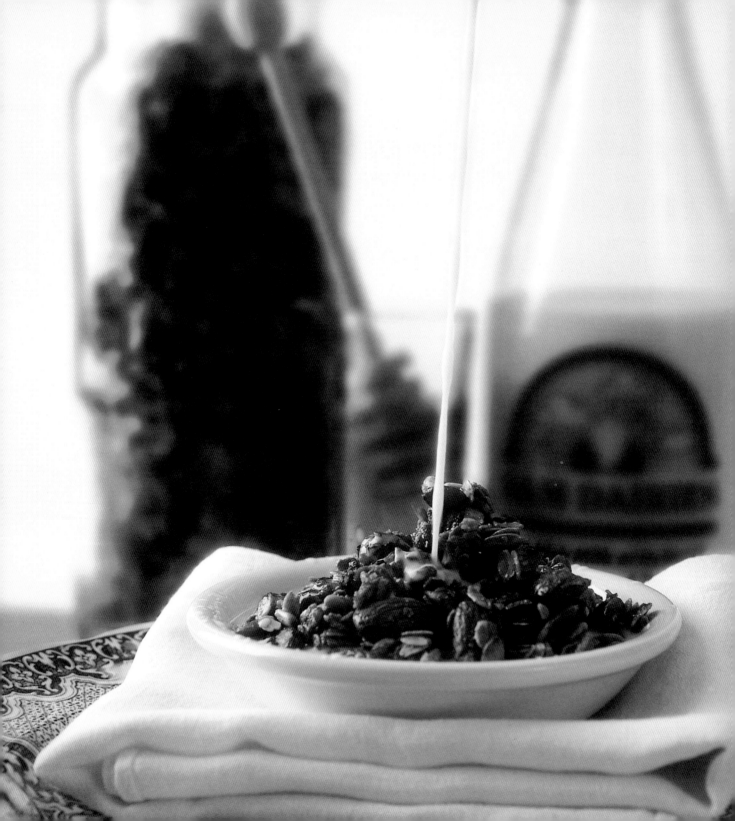

Two

BEAUTIFUL BREAKFASTS

Breakfast gets me going in the morning and I can't ever imagine leaving home without having eaten it, yet breakfast is the most commonly missed meal with people usually blaming their busy lifestyles, but all it takes is a little preparation to start your mornings on the right foot. I make granola and muesli most weekends so that I am always prepared for lack of time at breakfast.

It doesn't take long to make an omelette or boil an egg either and eggs contain lutein, an important antioxidant for eye health. Lutein is present in high concentrations in the macula and needs to be frequently replenished.

Always use the freshest eggs available. The Australian Egg Corporation recommends storing eggs in their original carton in the refrigerator as soon as possible after buying to maintain freshness. Keep them away from any pungent-smelling food items such as garlic, as eggs tend to absorb strong flavours.

When you are going to boil eggs remove them from the refrigerator and bring them to room temperature first as this will stop the shell from cracking due to sudden temperature change. Never boil eggs too rapidly as this can also crack the shell.

For perfect soft-boiled eggs, bring a saucepan of water to the simmer and using a spoon, gently add the room-temperature eggs to the water. Simmer for two minutes, then remove the saucepan from the heat and allow the eggs to sit in the hot water for a further two minutes. This will set the egg white and still keep the yolk runny.

If you're time-stressed make yourself a fruit smoothie. Smoothies don't take long to prepare and do an excellent job of recharging your body for whatever the day may bring.

Salt is optional in all recipes.

GRANOLA

100g (3½oz) brown sugar
150ml (5fl oz) honey
2 drops vanilla essence
2 tablespoons light olive oil
500g (1lb) rolled oats
70g (2½oz) shredded coconut

170g (5½oz) almonds, chopped
100g (3½oz) Brazil nuts, chopped
60g (2oz) sunflower seeds
60g (2oz) pumpkin seeds
Olive oil spray for greasing

Pre-heat oven to very slow, 120°C (250°F) Gas Mark 1.

Put the sugar, honey, vanilla and olive oil in a small saucepan and bring to the boil gradually. Remove from heat.

Mix the remaining ingredients together in a large bowl. Pour the hot honey mix over the oats mixture and stir thoroughly.

Place on a greased baking tray and bake for 40 minutes or until golden brown. Allow to cool. Serve with milk or orange juice.

Note: Cooking granola at such a low temperature will cook the oats and nuts fairly evenly; however you might need to stir once during cooking. Granola can be kept for up to four weeks in an airtight container.

ASPARAGUS, SPINACH AND GRUYERE OMELETTE

Serves 2

5 eggs
100ml (3fl oz) milk
50g (2oz) gruyere cheese, grated
1 cup baby spinach, washed, dried and
   roughly chopped

4 asparagus spears, woody ends
   removed and diced
Sea salt and freshly ground black pepper
Olive oil spray

Beat the eggs and milk in a small bowl, add the cheese, spinach and asparagus.
Season to taste with salt and pepper.
Heat a small frying pan and spray with olive oil. Pour half the egg mix into the pan
and cook on a medium to low heat for 4 minutes. Using a palette knife or egg flip
fold the omelette in half and gently slide on to a warm serving plate. Repeat with the
remaining mixture.

**Note: For a healthier option, use low-fat milk and reduced-fat tasty cheese can be
substituted for gruyere cheese.**

MY VERSION OF DR BIRCHER'S MUESLI

Serves 4

3 cups rolled oats
1½ cups (375ml/12fl oz) apple juice
1½ cups (375ml/12fl oz) orange juice
2 apples, grated
2 pears, grated

200ml (6fl oz) low-fat vanilla yoghurt
50g (2oz) slivered almonds
2 tablespoons honey
2 bananas
1 punnet blueberries

Soak the oats in the apple and orange juice in a bowl and refrigerate overnight. In the morning, fold through the apples, pears, yoghurt, almonds and half the honey. Serve topped with sliced banana and blueberries and drizzle with the remaining honey.

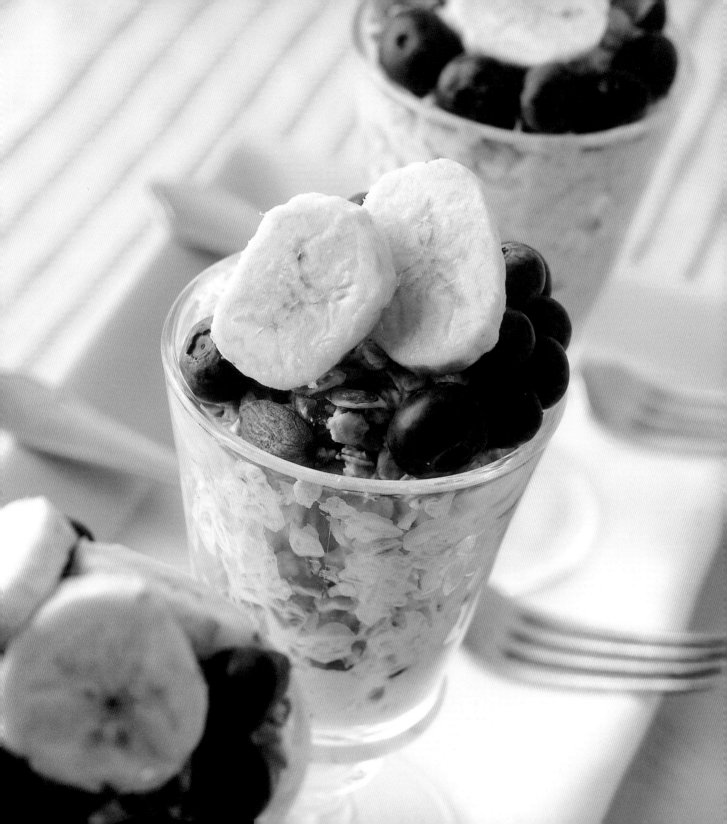

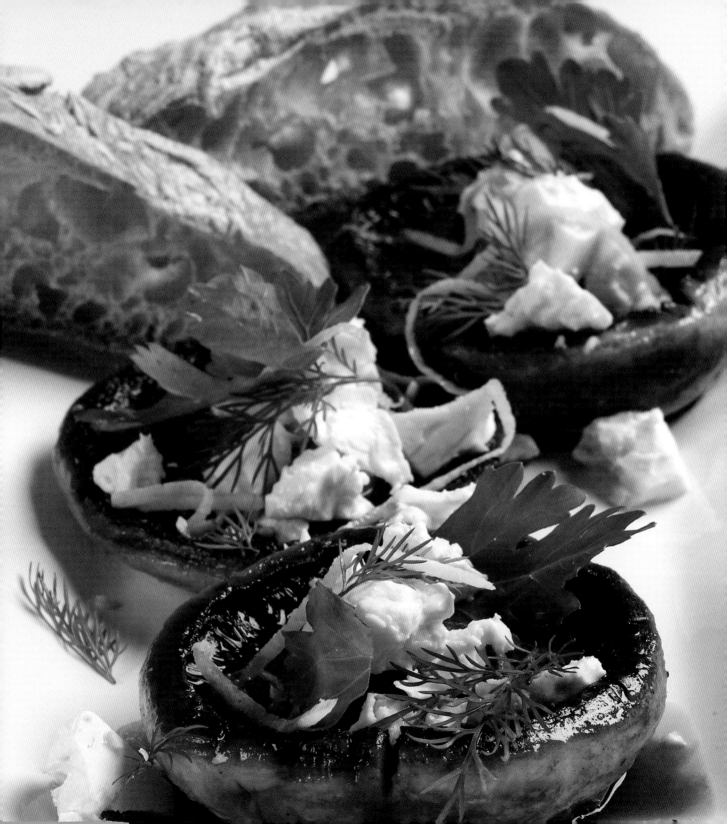

FIELD MUSHROOMS WITH SOFT HERBS, LEMON AND FETA

Serves 2

50g (2oz) butter

4 flat mushrooms, peeled and stalks
   trimmed

1 tablespoon balsamic vinegar

2 thick slices wood-fired sourdough
   bread, toasted

100g (3½oz) low-fat feta, crumbled

½ bunch parsley, washed and leaves
   picked

½ bunch dill, washed and leaves picked

Grated zest of 1 lemon

Freshly ground black pepper, to taste

Melt the butter in a frying pan. Add the mushrooms and cook for 3 minutes. Add the vinegar and simmer for another 3 minutes.

Remove the mushrooms (reserving the pan juices) and place them on the toast.

Spoon reserved pan juices over the mushrooms and top with the feta, parsley, dill, lemon zest and pepper.

Serve on warmed plates.

BREAKFAST SMOOTHIE

This healthy drink tastes delicious and doesn't take long to concoct. I like to use vanilla yoghurt because I prefer its sweeter taste.

2 cups (500ml/16fl oz) milk
1 tablespoon honey
2 tablespoons yoghurt, vanilla or natural
2 ripe bananas
Cinnamon powder

Puree all the ingredients in a blender until smooth. Pour into tall glasses and sprinkle cinnamon on top.

Note: For a healthier option use low-fat milk. Once bananas start to brown I cut them up into bite-size pieces and keep them in a zip-lock bag in the freezer so I can easily add them to my smoothies.

RAISIN TOAST WITH RICOTTA AND HONEYED FIGS

Serves 2

This is a wonderful late summer breakfast indulgence when fresh figs are in season.

2 tablespoons honey
100ml (3fl oz) low-fat fresh ricotta
½ teaspoon cinnamon powder
2 fresh figs, cut in half
2 slices raisin bread, thick cut

Heat the honey over low heat in a small saucepan.
Pour half the warmed honey into a bowl and mix in the ricotta and cinnamon.
Dip the cut side of the figs cut side up, into the honey that is still in the saucepan.
Cook the raisin bread and figs separately under the grill on a medium heat for 3 minutes.
Spread the ricotta mixture over the raisin toast, top with figs and any leftover honey and serve.

ALMOND AND BLUEBERRY PANCAKES WITH MAPLE SYRUP COMPOTE

Serves 4

1/3 cup (80ml/2½fl oz) maple syrup
100g (3½oz) blueberries, frozen or fresh
2 cups self-raising flour
¼ teaspoon baking powder
¼ cup flaked almonds

1 cup (250ml/8fl oz) low-fat milk
2 tablespoons honey
45g (1½oz) unsalted butter, melted,
2 eggs, lightly beaten
Extra butter for cooking

Make the maple syrup compote by heating the maple syrup in a small frying pan. Add half of the blueberries and gently simmer for 3 minutes or until the berries soften and the syrup becomes a deep purple colour.

Make a batter by sifting the flour and baking powder into a medium bowl. Mix in the almonds and make a well in the centre.

In another bowl, whisk together the milk, honey, butter and eggs and then pour this into the well of the dry mixture. Using a whisk, beat until there are no lumps and then gently mix in the remaining blueberries.

Heat a medium-sized frying pan, add a little butter and when melted, put 2 tablespoons of the batter into the pan, spread around and cook over a medium heat for 2 minutes or until the underside is golden.

Turn the pancake over and cook the other side then transfer to a plate and cover with a tea towel to keep warm.

Repeat with remaining batter, adding a little more butter to the pan if necessary.

Serve pancakes with the warm compote.

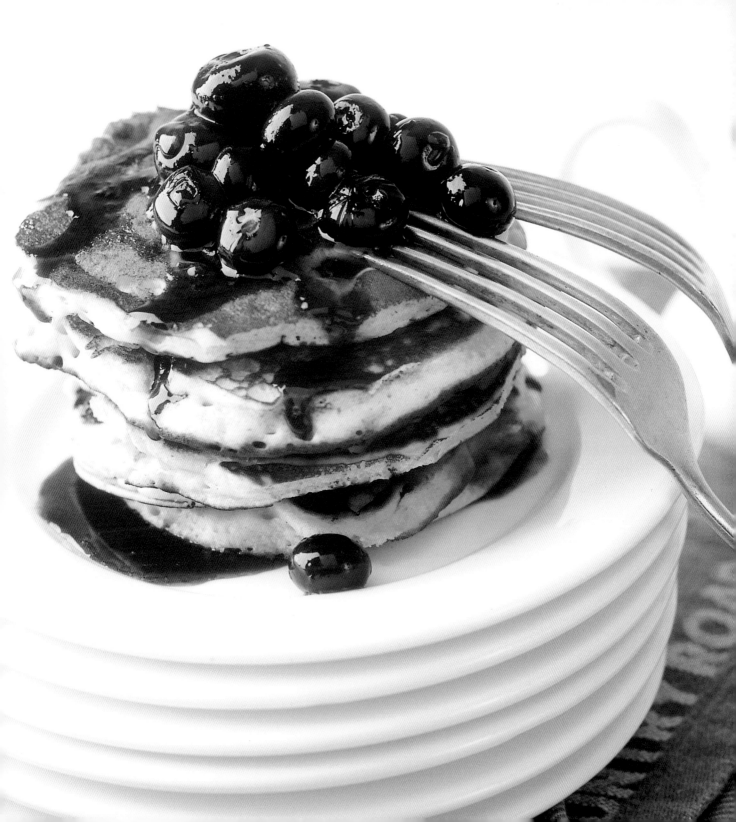

BANANA AND WALNUT LOAF

Makes 1 large loaf

This is fabulous served straight from oven with a little butter and strawberries when you feel you deserve a special treat. It's equally delicious served on its own.

Olive oil spray for greasing
450g (14½oz) plain flour
Sea salt, pinch
1 teaspoon nutmeg powder
1 teaspoon bicarbonate of soda

400g (13oz) caster sugar
5 eggs
250ml (8fl oz) light olive oil
1 cup walnut kernels, roughly chopped
4 ripe bananas, mashed

Pre-heat oven to moderate, 180°C (350°F) Gas Mark 4.
Spray a 31 x 9cm (12 x 3½ ins) loaf tin. In a large bowl, sift together the flour, salt, nutmeg and bicarbonate of soda.
Add the sugar, eggs and olive oil, stir until combined, then add the walnuts and bananas and mix together.
Pour into the loaf tin and cook for at least 1 hour.
Test if loaf is ready by inserting a skewer into the centre of the loaf. If it comes out clean the loaf is done. Turn out onto a wire rack.

Note: This loaf freezes well either whole or cut into smaller portions.

EGGS FLORENTINE

Serves 2

Hollandaise Sauce
100ml (3fl oz) white vinegar
4 egg yolks
250g (8oz) unsalted butter, melted
Juice of 1 lemon
Sea salt and freshly ground black pepper, to taste
1 tablespoon olive oil
1 clove garlic, minced
1 bunch spinach, washed and stalks removed
Sea salt and freshly ground black pepper, to taste
2 muffins, split and toasted
4 eggs, poached
Chives, chopped

To make the sauce, boil the vinegar until reduced by half. Allow to cool.
Using a double boiler, making sure the water in the bottom pot does not boil but just stays simmering on a low heat, pour the vinegar in to the top pot, add the yolks and whisk until ribbons begin to form and the egg mixture becomes thicker. Remove from the heat and continue to whisk while slowly adding the butter. Season to taste and add lemon juice. Cover with foil to keep warm until ready to use.
Heat the olive oil and sauté the garlic and spinach. Season. Drain excess liquid from the spinach and spoon evenly on to the muffins and top with eggs.
Drizzle with the hollandaise sauce and sprinkle with chives. Serve immediately.

Note: For a healthier option, omit the hollandaise sauce; you could sprinkle a little grated low-fat mozzarella cheese over the eggs instead.

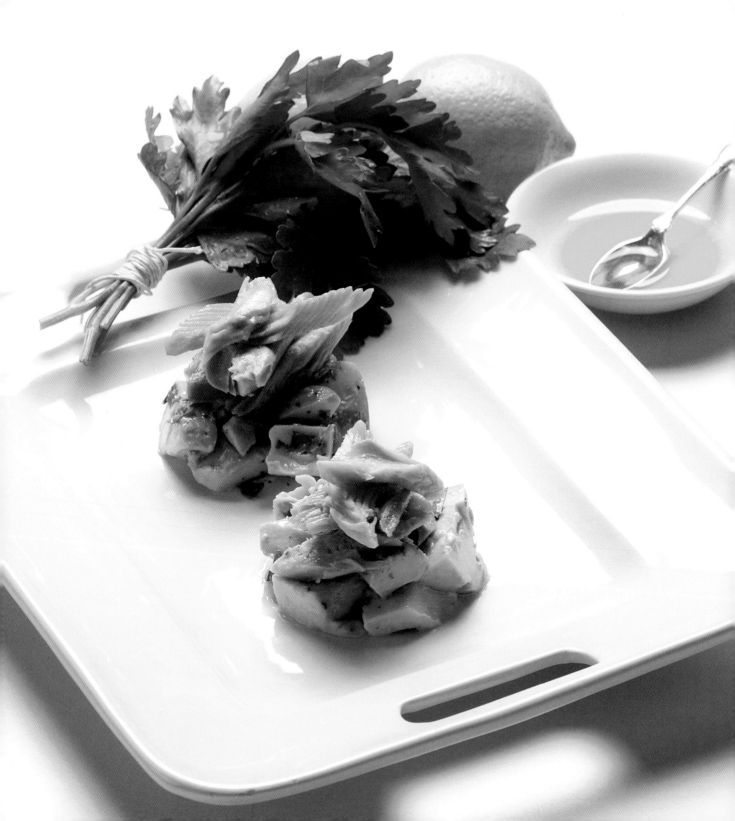

SMOKED TROUT WITH AVOCADO

Serves 2

200g (6½oz) smoked trout fillet
1 avocado
½ bunch flat leaf parsley, washed and
   chopped

Juice of 1 lemon
1 tablespoon extra virgin olive oil
Sea salt and freshly ground black pepper,
   to taste

Remove the skin from the trout and break the flesh into fairly large pieces and put to one side.

Peel the avocado and dice into a bowl with the parsley, lemon juice and the extra virgin olive oil and mix together. Season to taste with salt and pepper.

Put equal portions of the trout on a plate and serve with the avocado.

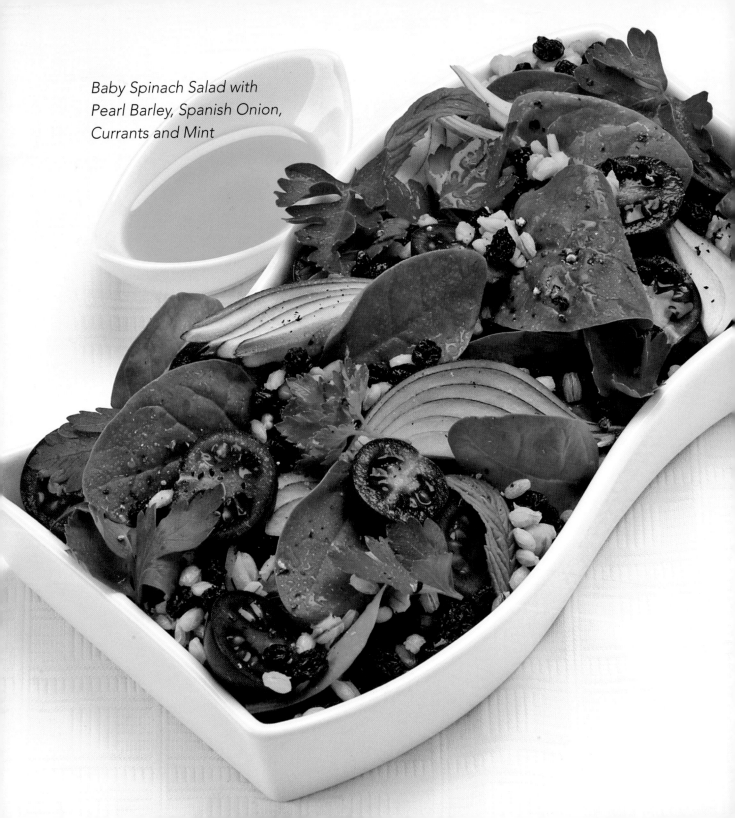

Baby Spinach Salad with Pearl Barley, Spanish Onion, Currants and Mint

Three

LEAFY GREENS

Spinach is the 'star' of this chapter. Many of the dishes are delicious on their own or can be served as an accompaniment to grilled (broiled) salmon, chicken or meat.

I was delighted to learn that spinach is one of the top vegetables for eye health because as far as I'm concerned baby spinach is one of the best and most versatile leafy greens of all. It can be sautéed, pureed, or simply served raw. Its flavour is not over-powering and it also makes an excellent base to any dish. Baby spinach also carries sauces well especially when it is used raw as sauces 'cling' to the leaves enabling the flavours to be spread throughout the dish.

It's important never to overcook spinach, something that's all too easy to do because it cooks so quickly. Eat spinach raw in salads, lightly cooked or steamed so it will not lose any of its beneficial qualities. You can freeze spinach but should always do so when it is fresh and the leaves are crisp. Store-bought packets of frozen spinach are a good substitute when fresh spinach is scarce.

Spinach is also one of the best sources of lutein which is essential for eye health and can help protect against macular degeneration. Lutein is also found in sweet corn, broccoli, asparagus, yellow squash and turnip greens. There are many varieties of spinach available these days and I use them in many of my recipes. As well as baby spinach, you also can choose from kale, silverbeet, gai larn, English spinach, chicory, chard and cavolo nero.

You may never look at spinach the same way again!

SPICED ENGLISH SPINACH WITH WATER CHESTNUTS

Serves 4 as a side dish

This is good served as a side dish with grilled (broiled) fish or roast lamb.

2 tablespoons turmeric powder
1 tablespoon cumin seeds
1 tablespoon poppy seeds
¼ cup (60ml/2floz) tamarind puree
  (see note)

½ cup (125ml/4floz) water
1 bunch English spinach, washed and
  roots removed
250g (8oz) tinned water chestnuts,
  drained and sliced

Gently dry roast the turmeric, cumin and poppy seeds in a large saucepan for two minutes. Add the tamarind puree and water and stir until combined then simmer on a low heat for 2 minutes. Add the spinach and chestnuts. Cook a further 3 minutes or until the spinach is a vibrant green and slightly wilted.

Note: Tamarind puree is available at Asian grocers and the Asian sections of large supermarkets. As tamarind is quite tart, a small amount of palm sugar may be added.

BABY SPINACH SALAD WITH PEARL BARLEY, SPANISH ONION, CURRANTS AND MINT

Serves 4 as a side dish

250g (8oz) pearl barley
100g (3½oz) baby spinach, washed and
  dried
100g (3½oz) currants
1 small Spanish onion, halved and sliced

1 punnet of cherry tomatoes, washed
  and halved
1 bunch mint, washed and leaves picked
1 bunch continental parsley, washed and
  leaves picked
1 tablespoon extra virgin olive oil

Boil the barley in 2 litres (3½ pints) of water for 30 minutes, drain and refresh in cold water.

Toss the barley with the spinach, currants, onion, cherry tomatoes, mint and parsley. Place in a serving bowl, drizzle with the extra virgin olive oil and serve (see picture page 48).

PLATE-SIZE SPINACH AND RICOTTA RAVIOLI WITH LA PUTTANESCA SAUCE

Serves 4

4 medium-sized vine-ripened tomatoes
1 cup rock salt (for baking tomatoes)
1 tablespoon light olive oil
400g (13oz) low-fat fresh ricotta
2 eggs, lightly beaten (for ravioli)
1 bunch English spinach, washed and finely chopped
2 tablespoons basil, chopped

Sea salt and freshly ground black pepper, to taste
400g (13oz) fresh lasagne sheets (cut into 8x16cm [6ins] squares)
1 egg, lightly beaten (for brushing)
800ml (1 1/3 pints) La Puttanesca Sauce (see next recipe)
2 tablespoons extra virgin olive oil

Pre-heat oven to moderately slow, 160°C (325°F) Gas Mark 3.

Place the tomatoes on a bed of rock salt in a baking dish, coat with olive oil and cook for 15 minutes. In a small bowl, combine the ricotta, eggs, spinach and basil. Season. Lay a lasagne sheet on a floured board, place 2 tablespoons of ricotta mixture on the sheet, brush the edges with beaten egg and cover with another lasagne sheet. Press the edges together to seal. Repeat until all the lasagne is used.

Bring a large pot of water to simmering point, gently put the ravioli in the water and cook for 6 minutes or until al dente.

Serve immediately with the hot Puttanesca Sauce and warm vine-ripened tomatoes.

Before serving drizzle the dish with the extra virgin olive oil.

Note: Fresh lasagne sheets are available at delicatessens or the refrigerated sections of supermarkets.

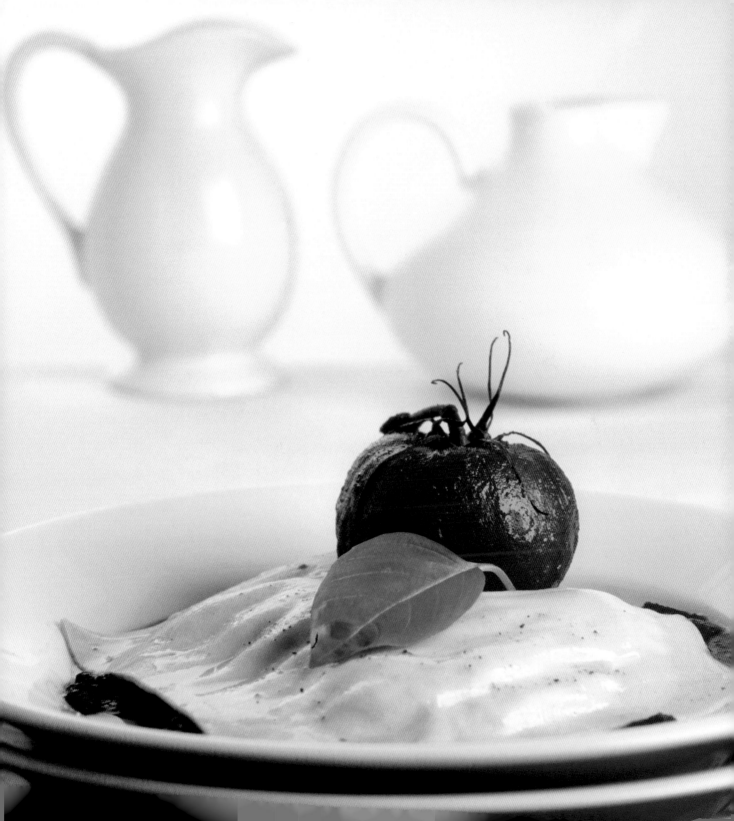

LA PUTTANESCA SAUCE

Makes 800ml (1¹/₃ pints)

¹/₃ cup (80ml/2½fl oz) light olive oil
2 cloves garlic, finely sliced
6 anchovy fillets
1 small red chilli, finely chopped
2 tablespoons capers, rinsed, dried and
   finely chopped

400g (13oz) tinned chopped tomatoes
1 tablespoon dried oregano
1 cup (250ml/8fl oz) white wine
½ cup pitted kalamata olives
Sea salt and ground black pepper

Heat the olive oil in a large frying pan, add the garlic, anchovy and chilli and cook until the anchovy fillets have dissolved.
Add the capers and tomatoes and simmer for 3 minutes. Add the oregano, wine and olives. Season to taste. Simmer gently on a low heat for at least 15 minutes.

SPRING GARDEN SALAD

Serves 4 as a side dish

500g (1lb) fresh peas
10 fresh baby corn, approximately 10cm
   (4ins) each
1 bunch spring onions, finely sliced
15 cherry tomatoes, washed and finely
   sliced
1 bunch basil, washed and dried, leaves
   picked

200g (6½oz) baby spinach, washed and
   dried
100g (3½oz) marinated feta
Grated zest of 1 lemon
2 tablespoons red wine vinegar
¼ cup (60ml/2fl oz) extra virgin olive oil
Sea salt and freshly ground black pepper

Shell the peas and lightly blanch with the corn in boiling water for 3 minutes. Drain and refresh in ice cold water.

Assemble the salad by combining the peas and corn with the spring onions, tomatoes, basil and spinach in a bowl.

Neatly arrange the salad on a serving platter and top with feta.

Make the dressing by combining the lemon zest, vinegar and extra virgin olive oil. Season to taste.

Drizzle the dressing over the salad and serve immediately.

Note: Persian feta is ideal for this dish and is available in delicatessens and large supermarkets.

GAI LARN (CHINESE BROCCOLI) WITH JAPANESE SESAME SAUCE

Serves 4 as a side dish

1 tablespoon white sesame seeds
1 tablespoon black sesame seeds
1 tablespoon olive oil
2 cloves garlic, minced

2 tablespoons oyster sauce
1/3 cup (80ml/2½ fl oz) mirin
1 bunch gai larn, washed and dried

Make the sauce by dry roasting the sesame seeds in a heavy–based frying pan on a low heat until slightly brown and fragrant.

Add the olive oil and garlic and continue to cook for a further 2 minutes. Add the oyster sauce and mirin and simmer for 3 minutes.

Trim the woody ends off the gai larn and cut into quarters, then blanch in boiling water for 4 minutes, and drain.

Arrange on a platter, pour over the sauce and serve.

Note: Mirin is a sweet rice-based wine used in Japanese cuisine. There are two types: hon mirin which contains about 14% alcohol and shin mirin, which has less than 1% alcohol. The flavour of both is the same. I use hon mirin but if you prefer less alcohol substitute with shin mirin. Both are available at Asian grocers and the Asian sections of large supermarkets.

FATOULA'S TRADITIONAL SILVERBEET PIE

Serves 6

Sea salt
1 bunch silverbeet, washed and stalks
   removed
5 eggs, lightly beaten
200g (6½oz) reduced-fat feta, crumbled
1 bunch green shallots (spring onions/
   scallions), washed and chopped

5 sprigs oregano, washed and chopped
10 basil leaves, washed and chopped
9 sheets packet filo pastry
200g (6½oz) unsalted butter, melted
Freshly ground black pepper, to taste
1 tablespoon cumin seeds

Pre-heat oven to moderate, 180°C (350°F) Gas Mark 4.

Bring a large saucepan of water to the boil, add a pinch of salt and the silverbeet and cook for 3 minutes. Drain and refresh in cold water.

Using a tea towel wring out the excess water from the silverbeet and roughly chop. Place in a bowl with the eggs, feta, shallots, oregano and basil and stir until combined. Pour the mixture into a 30 x 3cm (12 x 1½ ins) deep pie dish.

Unroll the pastry and place one piece on the pie dish allowing it to overlap the edges. Brush with the melted butter.

Put another layer of pastry on the pie dish again allowing it to overlap the edges and brush with the melted butter. Repeat this process 7 times.

Using a small sharp knife or kitchen scissors trim the edges of the pastry. To seal the pie press the edges with your finger. Sprinkle the last layer of pastry with a little pepper and the cumin seeds. Cook for 30 minutes. Serve warm.

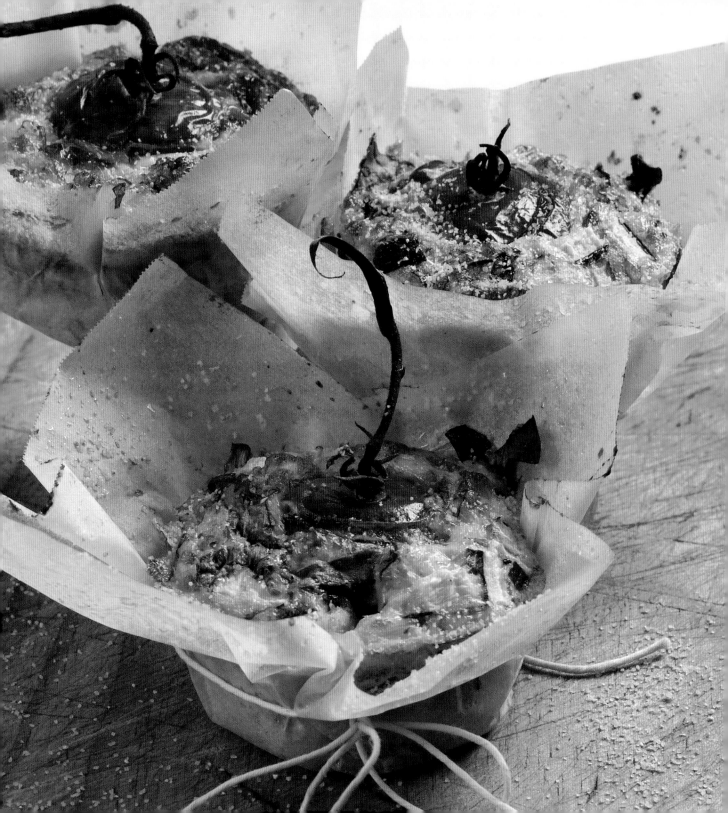

INDIVIDUAL ENGLISH SPINACH AND ZUCCHINI FRITTATAS

Makes 6 large frittatas

Olive oil spray
¼ cup polenta
8 eggs
1 cup (250ml/8fl oz) milk
3 zucchinis (courgettes), grated
2 tablespoons fresh parmesan cheese, grated

8 semi-dried tomatoes, chopped
4 basil leaves, washed and chopped
100g (3½oz) baby spinach, washed and finely chopped
Freshly ground black pepper and salt
6 cherry tomatoes, washed and dried

Pre-heat oven to moderate, 180°C (350°F) Gas Mark 4. Cut baking paper into squares and line muffin tin (100ml). Spray paper with olive oil and sprinkle with polenta so that all the sides of the muffin cups are coated.

Whisk the eggs and milk together then gently stir in the grated zucchini, parmesan, semi-dried tomatoes, basil, spinach and a little pepper and salt.

Fill the muffin cups with the mixture, top with a cherry tomato and cook for 20 minutes.

Frittatas can be served hot or cold.

Note: For a healthier option, use low-fat milk. Packet or tinned parmesan cheese can be substituted but fresh will give much better flavour. If you don't have 100ml (3fl oz) muffin cups, make smaller frittatas in a 12 cup muffin tin and reduce the cooking time by 5 minutes.

BABY SPINACH AND STRAWBERRY SALAD

Serves 4 as a side dish

200g (6½oz) baby spinach leaves, washed and dried

1 punnet strawberries, washed and tops removed

3 sprigs tarragon, stalks removed and leaves chopped

8 basil leaves, washed and chopped

¼ cup flaked almonds

1 tablespoon pumpkin seeds

1 tablespoon honey

¼ cup (60ml/2fl oz) balsamic vinegar

¼ cup (60ml/2fl oz) extra virgin olive oil

Sea salt

Place the spinach, strawberries, herbs, almonds and pumpkin seeds in a large bowl. Make dressing by whisking together the honey, vinegar, olive oil and a pinch of salt. Drizzle over the salad and serve immediately.

ICEBERG LETTUCE AND PEA SALAD

Serves 4 as a side dish

¼ cup (60ml/2fl oz) extra virgin olive oil
1 tablespoon seeded mustard
Juice of 2 lemons
1 cup frozen baby peas
½ iceberg lettuce, washed and torn into bite-size pieces
1 bunch mint, leaves washed and picked

To make dressing, whisk the olive oil, mustard and lemon juice together in a bowl until combined.
Blanch the peas in boiling water for 30 seconds, drain and refresh in ice cold water.
Toss the lettuce, peas and mint leaves together in a bowl, add the dressing and serve.

SORREL AND POTATO SOUP

Serves 4

1 tablespoon olive oil
1 large onion, roughly chopped
2 cloves garlic, minced
500g (1lb) pontiac potatoes, roughly
  chopped
2 leeks, washed and chopped
2 bunches sorrel, washed and roots
removed, roughly chopped
1 bunch basil, washed, leaves picked and
  roughly chopped
1 litre (1¾ pints) chicken stock
Sea salt and freshly ground black pepper
Mascarpone

Heat the olive oil in a large saucepan and sauté the onions, garlic, potatoes, leeks, sorrel and basil for 4 minutes.
Add the chicken stock and simmer for 30 minutes. Remove from the heat and puree in a blender.
Season to taste with salt and pepper and serve with a dollop of mascarpone and warm crusty bread.

Note: Homemade chicken stock is best but reduced-salt packet stock can be substituted. For a healthier option, omit the mascarpone.

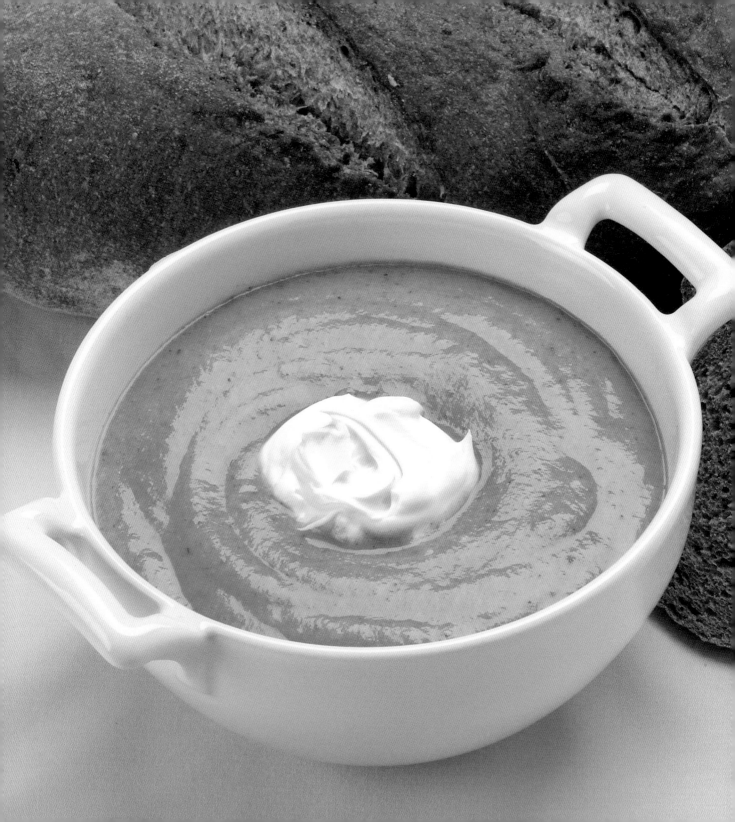

BABY SPINACH, YELLOW BEETROOT AND CANNELLINI SALAD

Serves 4 as a side dish

4 yellow baby beetroot
200g (6½oz) tinned cannellini beans
100g (3½oz) baby spinach, washed and
    dried
1 bunch flat leaf parsley, washed and
    leaves picked

1 bunch dill, washed and leaves picked
1 Spanish onion, sliced
Sea salt
Extra virgin olive oil
Juice of 1 lemon

Place the unpeeled beetroot in cold water then bring to the boil and cook for 5 minutes or until tender. Drain and refresh in cold water.

Peel and cut the beetroot in half.

Drain the beans and rinse with cold water. Place them in a large bowl with the beetroot, spinach, herbs and onion.

Season to taste with salt.

Drizzle with the extra virgin olive oil and lemon juice and serve.

ENGLISH SPINACH AU GRATIN

Serves 4 as a side dish

Sea salt
1 bunch English spinach, washed and stems removed
100g (3½oz) reduced-fat sour cream
50g (2oz) gruyere cheese, grated
1 tablespoon wholemeal breadcrumbs

Pre-heat oven to moderate, 180°C (350°F) Gas Mark 4.
Blanch the spinach in salted boiling water for 2 minutes then drain and refresh in cold water. Place in a tea towel and wring out any excess water.
Mix with the sour cream in a bowl until the leaves are lightly coated. Arrange in a medium ceramic baking dish, sprinkle with gruyere cheese and breadcrumbs.
Cook for 10 minutes or until golden brown and serve.

Note: For a healthier option, use reduced-fat tasty cheese.

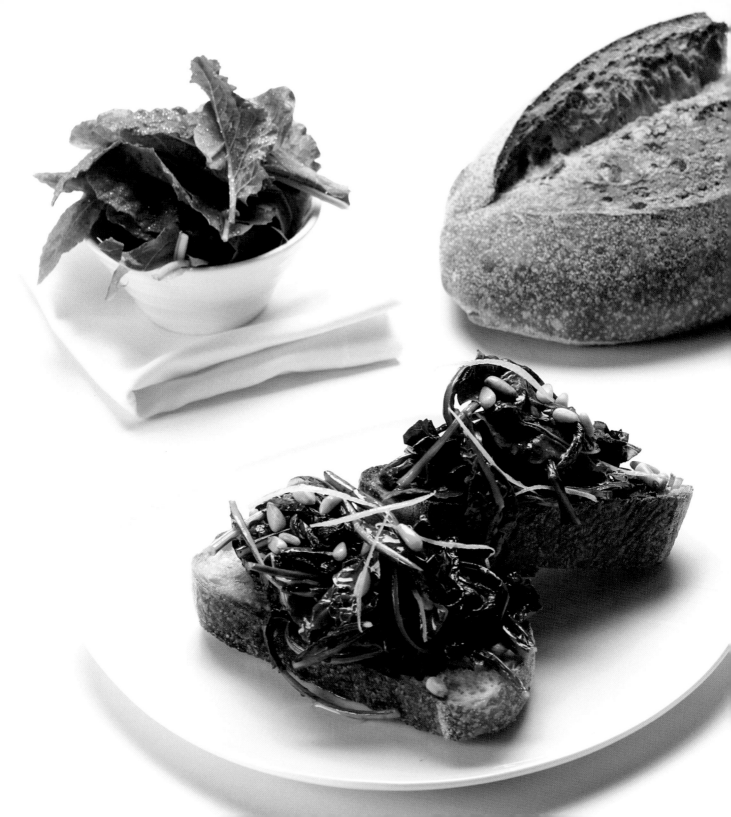

CAVOLO NERO (ITALIAN SPINACH) ON GARLIC SOURDOUGH TOPPED WITH PINE NUTS

Serves 4

1 loaf sourdough bread, day old is best
2 tablespoons olive oil
3 cloves garlic, thinly sliced
100g (3½oz) cavolo nero leaves, washed and dried
Grated zest of 1 lemon
Pine nuts, dry roasted
Sea salt and freshly ground black pepper

Pre-heat oven to moderate, 180°C (350°F) Gas Mark 4.
Cut 4 slices of bread approximately 7cm (2¾ins) thick and brush with 1 tablespoon of olive oil.
Sprinkle half the garlic on the bread, put on a baking tray and cook for 7 minutes.
Heat the remaining oil in a medium-sized saucepan, sauté the cavolo nero for 3 minutes or until wilted, add the rest of the garlic and the lemon zest and season to taste with salt and pepper.
Serve on the crispy baked bread and sprinkle with pine nuts.

Note: Dry roast pine nuts in a heavy based frying pan on low heat.

FENNEL AND ORANGE SALAD

Serves 4 as a side dish

1 large fennel bulb, washed and dried
3 navel oranges, peeled and sliced
4 basil leaves, washed and chopped
1/3 cup pumpkin seeds, dry roasted
Extra virgin olive oil

Pick the leafy tops from the fennel, remove the tough outer layers and finely slice the bulb. Place the slices in ice cold water for 20 minutes.
Arrange the sliced oranges on a platter, top with the sliced fennel bulb, basil and leafy fennel tops.
Sprinkle with the pumpkin seeds, dress with the extra virgin olive oil and serve.

Note: Dry roast pumpkin seeds in a heavy based frying pan on low heat.

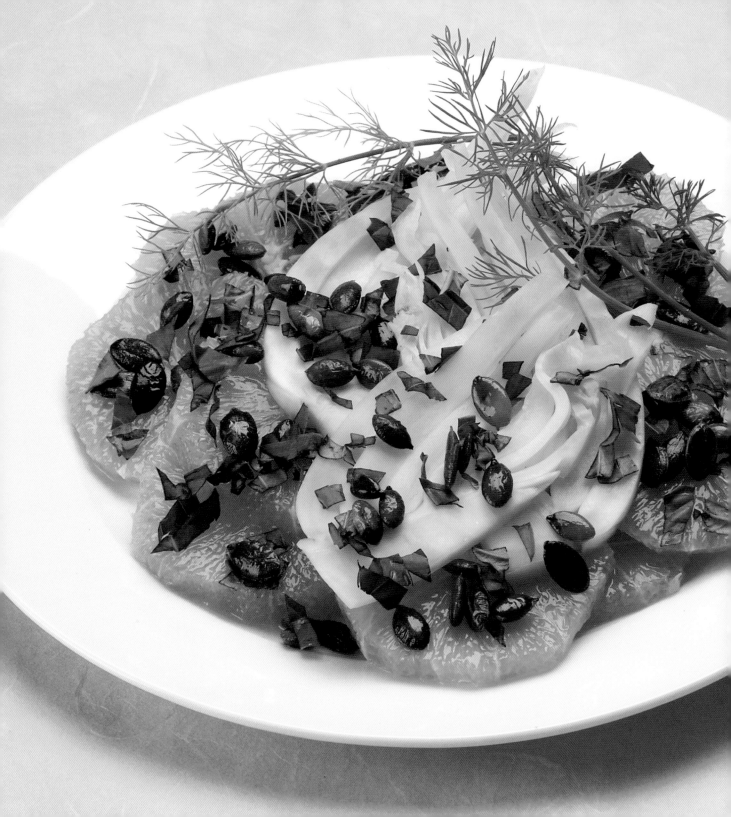

SILVERBEET AND BLUE CHEESE SOUP

Serves 6

1 tablespoon olive oil
1 brown onion, chopped
2 cloves garlic, chopped
1 bunch silverbeet, washed and stalks
   removed
1 cup (250ml/8fl oz) white wine

1 litre (1¾ pints) chicken stock
1 litre (1¾ pints) water
Sea salt and freshly ground black pepper,
   to taste
200ml (6fl oz) cream
100g (3½oz) blue cheese

Heat the olive oil in a large saucepan and sauté the onions, garlic and silverbeet until soft. Add the white wine, chicken stock and water and simmer for 30 minutes.
Remove from the heat and puree, using a blender.
Add the cream and season to taste with salt and pepper.
Sprinkle with a little crumbled blue cheese and serve with warm crusty bread.

Note: Be careful when seasoning soup with salt as blue cheese tends to be quite salty. Homemade is best but reduced-salt packet stock can be substituted. For a healthier option, omit the cream or substitute reduced-fat cream.

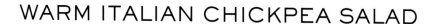

WARM ITALIAN CHICKPEA SALAD

Serves 4 as a side dish

200g (6½oz) tinned chickpeas
3 baby eggplants (aubergines), tops
   removed and cut into quarters
2 green zucchinis (courgettes), tops
   removed and cut into quarters
1 punnet cherry tomatoes

1 Spanish onion, quartered
4 cloves garlic, left whole
6 basil leaves, washed and torn
Olive oil
Sea salt and freshly ground black pepper
2 tablespoons balsamic vinegar

Pre-heat oven to moderately slow, 160°C (325°F) Gas Mark 3.

Drain and wash the chickpeas in cold water. Scatter all the vegetables, except the chickpeas, in a large baking dish.

Add the garlic and basil, coat with olive oil, season to taste with salt and pepper and cook for 45 minutes.

Toss the chickpeas through the hot vegetables, arrange on a serving platter, drizzle with the vinegar and serve.

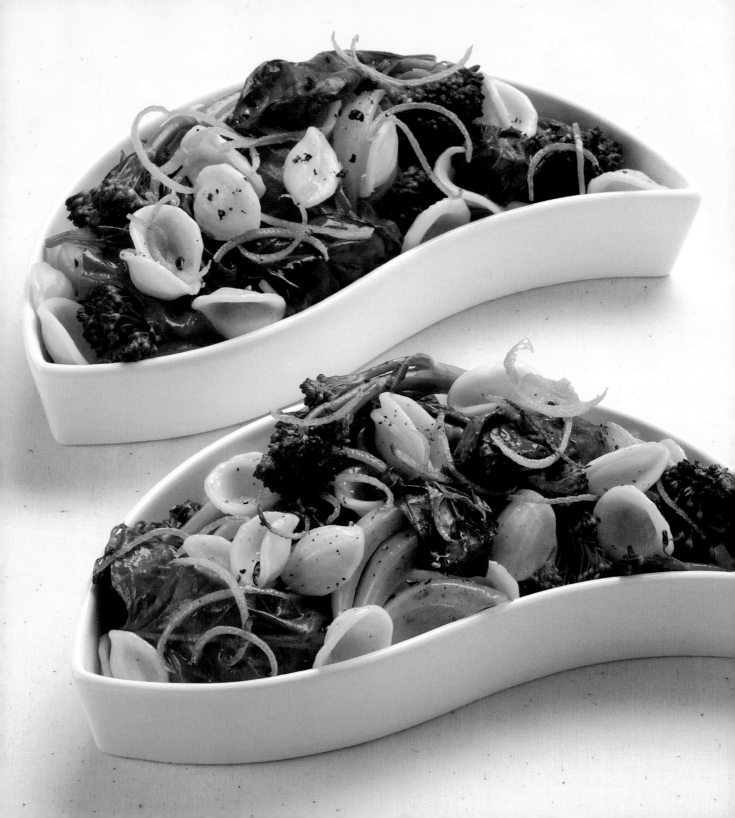

ORECCHIETTE WITH ENGLISH SPINACH, BROCCOLINI, LEMON AND GARLIC

Serves 4

300g (9½oz) orecchiette pasta
1 bunch broccolini, washed and woody
   ends trimmed
2 tablespoons olive oil
1 onion, diced
2 cloves garlic, sliced
Grated zest of 1 lemon

½ bunch basil, leaves washed and
   chopped
12 English spinach leaves, washed and
   stems removed
Best quality extra virgin olive oil
Sea salt and freshly ground black pepper

Bring a large saucepan of salted water to the boil, add the orecchiette and cook for 15 minutes or until al dente. Drain and refresh with cold water.

Boil the broccolini in a saucepan for 4 minutes, remove and slice into small pieces.

Heat the olive oil in a large frying pan and cook the onion, garlic and broccolini for 5 minutes or until tender.

Add the orecchiette, stir until combined and then add the lemon zest, basil and spinach.

Season to taste with salt and pepper, drizzle with the extra virgin olive oil and serve immediately.

Note: A head of broccoli can be substituted for broccolini.

SAUTÉED SILVERBEET WITH MUSTARD SEED, CUMIN AND CHILLI TOPPED WITH COCONUT

Serves 4 as a side dish

2 tablespoons olive oil
1 brown onion, diced
2 cloves garlic, finely sliced
1 small chilli, seeds removed and finely
   sliced
1 tablespoon mustard seeds

2 tablespoons black sesame seeds
2 tablespoons fennel seeds
1 bunch silverbeet, washed, stalks
   removed and leaves shredded
Sea salt
¼ cup shredded coconut, toasted

Heat the olive oil in a large saucepan and sauté onions and garlic for 2 minutes or until translucent.
Add the chilli, mustard, sesame and fennel seeds and cook for a further 2 minutes.
Add the shredded silverbeet and toss until coated in spices.
Season to taste with salt. Sprinkle with toasted coconut and serve immediately.

CHARD, BASIL AND PEANUTS

Serves 4 as a side dish

1 tablespoon olive oil

1 brown onion, diced

2 cloves garlic, minced

1 teaspoon fresh ginger, minced

1 teaspoon yellow mustard seeds

1 tablespoon turmeric powder

3 ripe tomatoes, washed and diced

1 bunch basil, leaves picked, washed and chopped

800g (1lb 10oz) baby chard leaves, washed and dried

2 tablespoons salted peanuts, crushed

Heat the olive oil in a saucepan, then cook the onion, garlic, ginger, mustard seeds and turmeric for 3 minutes or until aromatic.

Add the tomatoes, basil, chard and peanuts and stir until the chard and basil leaves start to wilt.

Serve immediately.

Note: Chard is a pretty leafy green with lightly purple leaves that have bright red veins. It is usually available at greeng

MISO BROTH WITH UDON NOODLES AND WAKAME

Serves 4

1 litre (1¾ pints) water
1 tablespoon miso paste
2 tablespoons reduced-salt soy sauce
50g (2oz) wakame (seaweed), dried
2 baby bok choy (pak choi), washed and cut in quarters

200g (6½oz) udon noodles
100g (3½oz) silken tofu, diced
4 sprigs coriander (cilantro), leaves washed and picked
4 sprigs mint, leaves washed and picked

To make the broth bring a saucepan of water to the boil, add the miso paste and soy sauce and mix together thoroughly. Put to one side.

Put the wakame and bok choy in a bowl, cover with boiling water and stand for 4 minutes. Drain and refresh under cold water.

Bring a large saucepan of water to the boil, add the noodles and cook for 5 minutes. Drain and refresh in cold water.

Re-boil the broth, divide the noodles, wakame, bok choy, and tofu into four bowls and cover with the broth.

Sprinkle with the coriander and mint leaves and serve.

Note: Bok choy (pak choi) is available from Asian grocers, supermarkets and is a small, green Chinese vegetable.

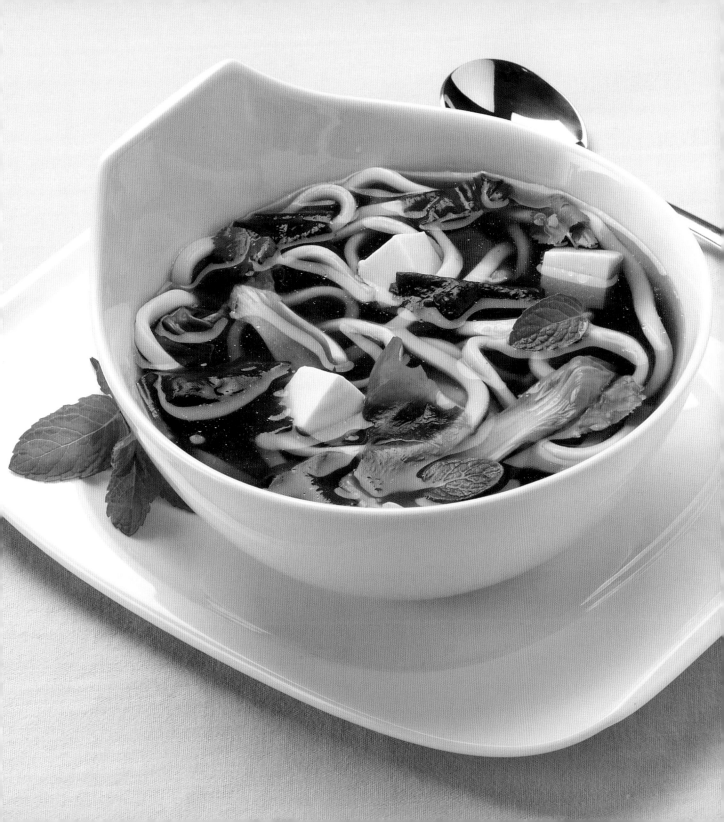

FRENCH BEAN SALAD WITH SALSA VERDE

Serves 4 as a side dish

1 tablespoon capers
1 bunch flat leaf parsley, washed and leaves picked
3 anchovies
2 tablespoons extra virgin olive oil
100g (3½oz) green beans, washed and tops removed
100g (3½oz) yellow beans, washed and tops removed
100g (3½oz) broad beans, shelled

To make the salsa verde, puree the capers, parsley, anchovies and olive oil in a food processor until smooth.

Blanch the beans together in boiling water for 4 minutes, refresh in iced cold water, toss into the salsa verde and serve.

QUICK WAYS WITH ICEBERG LETTUCE

- Break large pieces of lettuce in a bowl. Add a handful of watercress leaves, a shave of fresh parmesan cheese and some sliced pear. Dress with extra virgin olive oil and a squeeze of lemon. Sprinkle with chopped Brazil nuts.

- Cut lettuce into wedges. Make a dressing by pureeing blue cheese and olive oil together. Drizzle over the lettuce. Crumble a little blue cheese on top.

- Tear the lettuce leaves into large pieces, toss with parsley leaves, dill, chervil, chives, basil and handful of watercress. Dress with lemon juice and extra virgin olive oil plus a sprinkle of sea salt.

- Skin and slice a couple of oranges. Toss with lettuce leaves and basil leaves. Dress with extra virgin olive oil. I sometimes add a few kalamata olives.

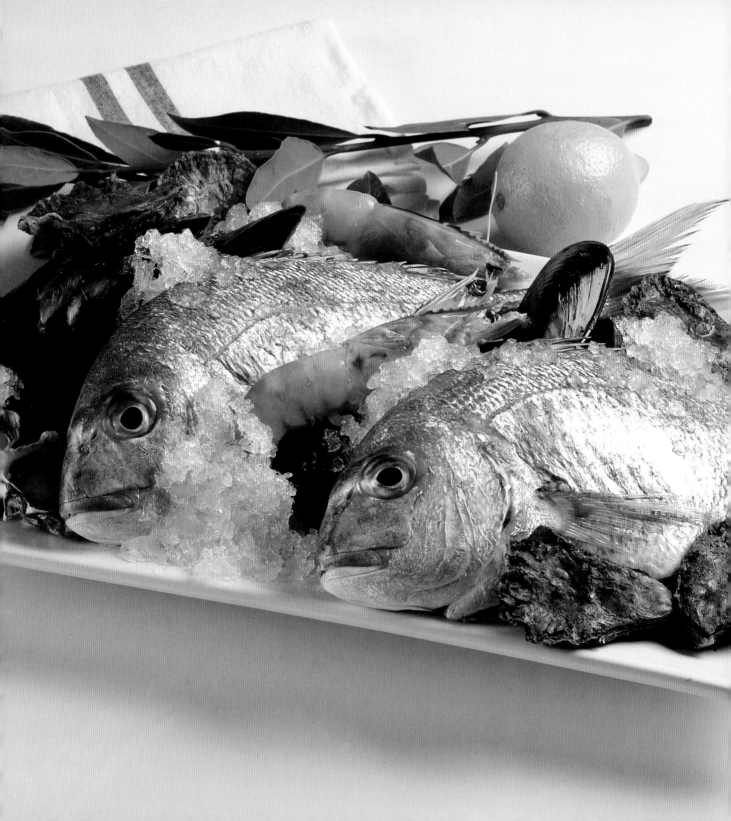

Four

FROM THE OCEAN

My mother used to buy whole snapper from our local beach fishermen and would stuff the fish with sliced onions and tomatoes and serve it with fresh lemons from our tree in the garden and a big bowl of homemade chips. She declared that it was a meal fit for a king. Indeed it was!

My favourite fish is sashimi grade yellowfin tuna which I eat raw, thinly sliced and dipped in a little soy sauce mixed with a smear of wasabi.

Fish, particularly oily varieties such as salmon, sardines, and trout, is an excellent source of omega-3 fatty acids, which are good for eye health. Seafood contains zinc which is also necessary for your eye health. Oysters are the best source of zinc with 100g (3½oz) of oysters providing approximately 48mg of zinc.

Always buy the freshest fish possible. Look for a fish with plump clear eyes, firm flesh, tight scales and bright red gills. If you can't get fresh, use frozen or tinned fish, preferably in spring water or brine. It doesn't matter which way you eat it, fish is good for your health. Fresh salmon freezes particularly well and you can buy a few extra pieces and put them in the freezer if getting to the fishmonger on a regular basis is difficult.

Versatile fish can be a simple meal or a lavish feast.

WHITE ANCHOVIES
AND GREEN OLIVE TAPENADE ON A CROUTON

Serves 4 as an entrée

These can also be served as nibbles with drinks. White anchovies have a far more delicate flavour than regular anchovies as they are not as salty and are softer in texture. They are usually available already marinated at delicatessens.

1 sesame seed breadstick
50g (2oz) unsalted butter, melted
250g (8oz) pitted green olives
100ml (3fl oz) light olive oil
2 cloves garlic Juice of 1 lemon Extra virgin olive oil
16 white anchovies
Freshly ground black pepper

Pre-heat oven to moderate, 180°C (350°F) Gas Mark 4.
Cut the bread stick into 8 slices and lightly brush with butter. Bake for 7–8 minutes or until golden brown. Remove from oven and cool.
Make the tapenade by blending the olives, extra virgin olive oil, garlic and lemon juice in a food processor. Neatly spoon a teaspoonful of tapenade on each crouton, top with two white anchovies, drizzle with a little extra virgin olive oil and sprinkle with a little pepper.

OYSTERS WITH ESCHALOT DRESSING

Serves 2

Oysters are best served in the shell; however they can be served in ceramic Chinese spoons as an impressive canapé.

¹/₃ cup (80ml/2½ fl oz) fish sauce
¹/₃ cup (80ml/2½ fl oz) lime juice
1 bird's-eye chilli, seeds removed, finely sliced
1 tablespoon palm sugar
1 eschallot, washed and diced

1 Lebanese cucumber, washed and finely sliced
24 oysters
½ bunch Thai basil , washed and leaves picked, finely chopped

Make the dressing by combining the fish sauce, lime juice, chilli, palm sugar and eschallot in a small saucepan. Simmer for 4 minutes or until palm sugar has dissolved. Allow to cool.

Keep oysters in the half shell, top with the cucumber and basil. Drizzle over the dressing and serve immediately.

Note: Thai basil is available at most greengrocers. It has a slight purple tinge to its leaf and stem and its strong sweet aniseed taste is perfect for seafood.

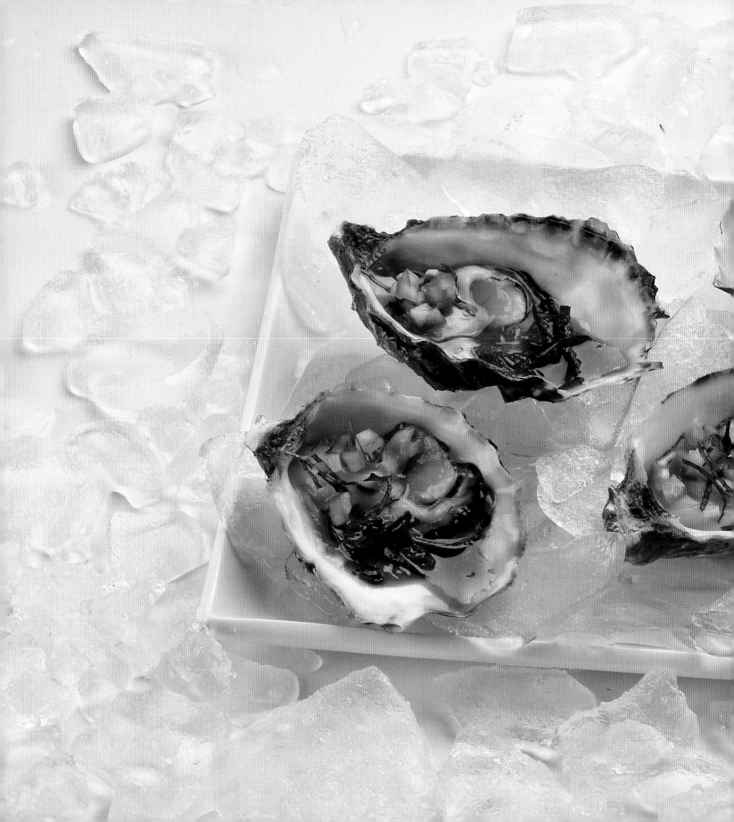

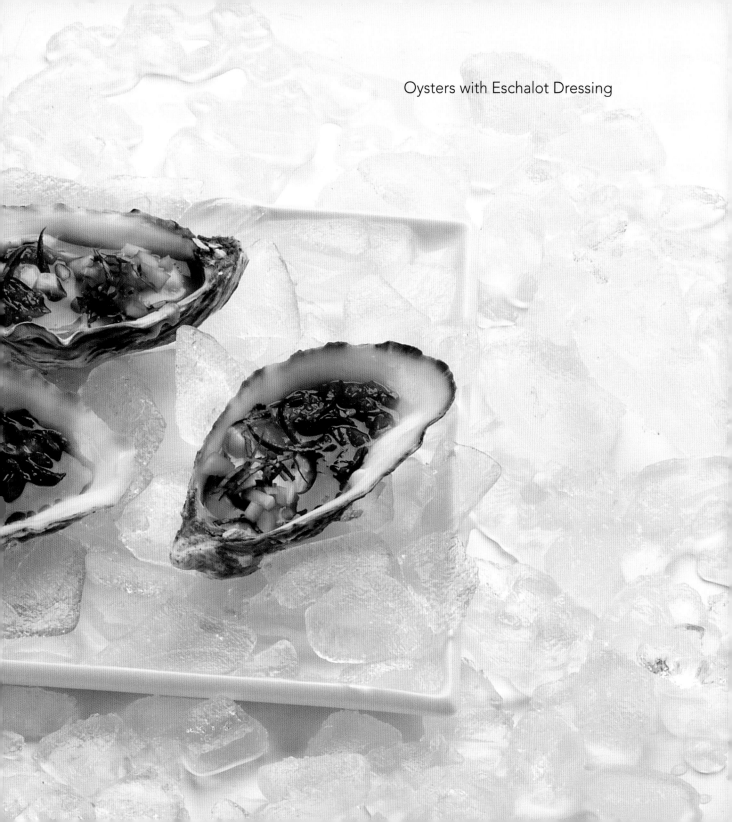

Oysters with Eschalot Dressing

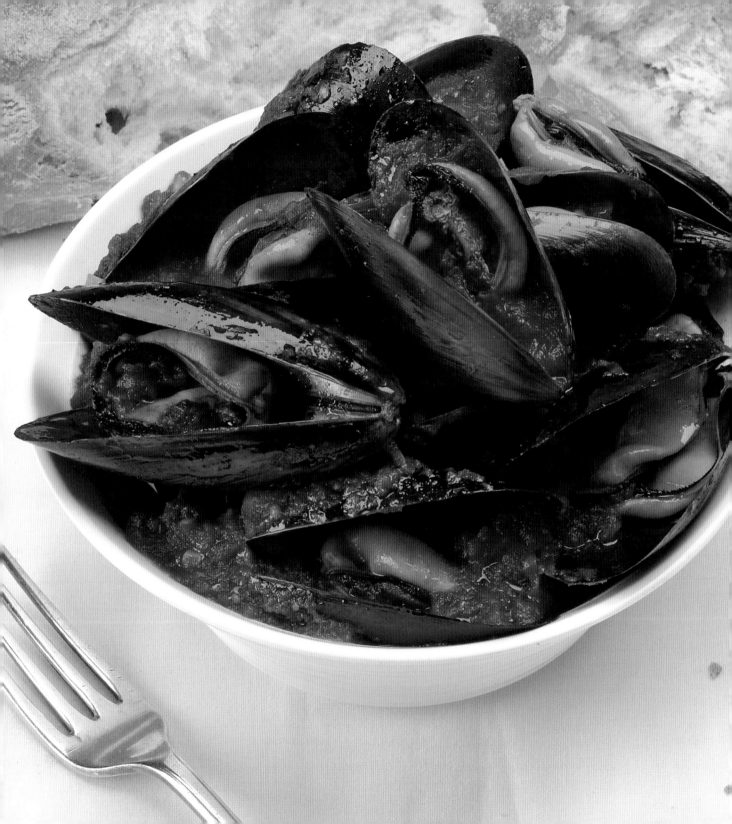

BLACK MUSSELS IN SPICY TOMATO SAUCE

Serves 4 as an entrée, or 2 as a main course

1kg (2lbs) black mussels (clams)
50ml (1½fl oz) olive oil
1 large onion, diced
4 cloves garlic, minced
1½ teaspoons hot smoked Spanish paprika powder
250ml (8fl oz) dry white wine
400g (13oz) tinned diced tomatoes

Heat the olive oil in a large saucepan and gently cook the onion, garlic and paprika until soft.

Add the mussels, white wine and tomatoes and cover the saucepan for 6–7 minutes or until all the mussels open.

Spoon the mussels into four warmed bowls, pour over the sauce and serve with crusty bread.

Note: Mussels should be bought live. When buying mussels make sure the shells are not cracked or tightly closed but snap shut when tapped—this shows they're still alive. Eat within 3 days. To clean a mussel grab the protruding clump of hairs called the 'beard' and pull with a sharp downward tug. Scrub the shells to remove excess grit or weed and rinse well.

TROUT, BLOOD ORANGE AND RADICCHIO SALAD

Serves 2

1 whole smoked trout, skinned, bones removed

1 head radicchio, washed, dried and torn into bite-size pieces

6 caperberries, cut in halves (optional)

2 blood oranges, skin removed, cut to bite size

2 tablespoons white balsamic vinegar

¼ cup (60ml/2fl oz) extra virgin olive oil

25g (1oz) salmon roe pearls

Sea salt and freshly ground black pepper

To prepare trout, use a knife to remove the head and tail and carefully peel the skin away from the flesh. Run a knife along the spine of the fish and the flesh will lift from bone with ease. Break flesh into bite-size pieces.

Assemble the salad by tossing pieces of trout and radicchio with the caperberries and blood orange.

Make the dressing by combining vinegar, extra virgin olive oil and salmon roe pearls in a bowl. Season to taste with salt and pepper and gently mix together.

Gently dress salad with the dressing and serve immediately.

Note: Salmon roe pearls are fragile so be careful not to damage them while mixing.

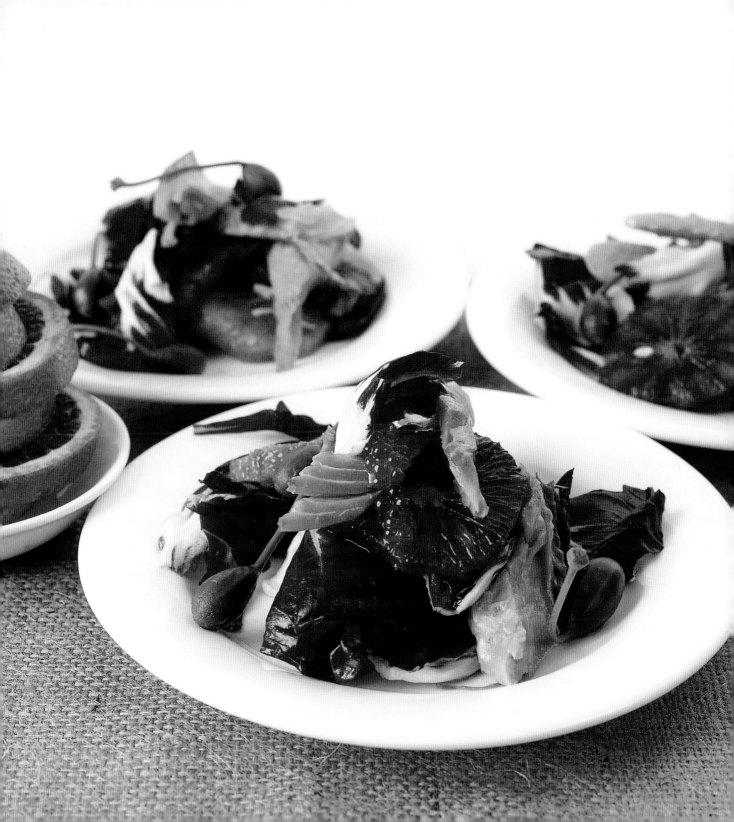

SAFFRON AND TOMATO BOUILLABAISSE

Serves 6

1 tablespoon olive oil
2 large onions, diced
3 cloves garlic, diced
4 tomatoes, washed, diced
12 black mussels (clams), scrubbed and beard removed
2 raw blue swimmer crabs, lungs and roe removed

200g (3½oz) salmon fillets, skin removed, diced large
6 baby octopus, cleaned and cut in halves
12 green prawns (shrimp), body peeled, heads and tails left on
15 threads saffron

4 sprigs tarragon
750ml (24fl oz) white wine
750ml (24fl oz) fish stock
2 fennel bulbs, washed, trimmed and cut in quarters
1 lemons, quartered for serving

Heat the olive oil in a large saucepan and sauté the onions, garlic, tomatoes, mussels and crabs on a medium heat for approximately 5 minutes or until crab shells have just turned pink. Add the salmon, octopus and prawns. In a separate saucepan bring the white wine, stock, saffron, tarragon sprigs and fennel to the simmer for 10 minutes. Pour the hot stock over the seafood and continue to simmer for a further 10 minutes. Serve immediately with warm crusty bread and lemon quarters.

Note: Mussels should be bought live. When buying mussels make sure the shells are not cracked or tightly closed but snap shut when tapped—this shows they're still alive. Eat within 3 days. To clean a mussel grab the protruding clump of hairs called the 'beard' and pull with a sharp downward tug. Scrub the shells to remove excess grit or weed and rinse well.

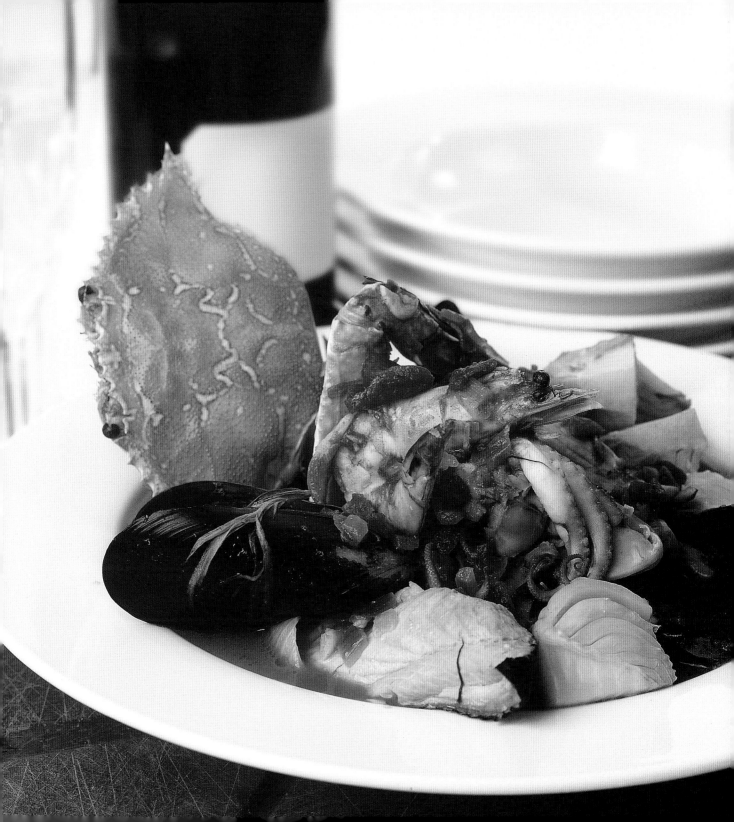

GRILLED SARDINES WITH LEMON, THYME AND PINE NUTS

Serves 4 as an entrée, or 2 as a main course

⅓ cup (80ml/2½fl oz) extra virgin olive oil
Juice and grated zest of 4 lemons
¼ loaf day-old bread
½ bunch thyme, washed and leaves
   removed
2 tablespoons pine nuts

Sea salt
12 fresh sardine fillets
1 bunch rocket, washed and stalks
   trimmed

Pre-heat oven to moderately hot, 200°C (400°F) Gas Mark 5.

Make a vinaigrette by whisking the olive oil and lemon juice in a small jug, add half lemon zest.

Place the bread, thyme, pine nuts, a pinch of salt and remaining lemon zest in a food processor and lightly pulse for 3 seconds to make breadcrumbs.

Line a baking tray with baking paper.

Place the sardine fillets, flesh side up, on the tray and sprinkle with the breadcrumbs.

Cook for 10 minutes and serve on a bed of rocket, drizzled with the lemon vinaigrette.

Note: Ask your fishmonger for sardine fillets. The head and all bones will be removed.

SEARED PEPPERED TUNA NICOISE SALAD

Serves 2

1 bunch parsley, leaves washed and
    picked
6 anchovy fillets
1/3 cup (80ml/2½ fl oz) extra virgin olive
    oil
Juice of 3 lemons
50g (2oz) green beans
50g (2oz) yellow beans

2 eggs, soft boiled
2 x 200g (6½oz) yellow fin tuna fillets
¼ cup freshly ground black pepper
Sea salt
2 tablespoons light olive oil
1 cup baby spinach, washed and dried
¼ cup green Sicilian olives
¼ cup kalamata olives

Make the dressing by putting the parsley, anchovies, extra virgin olive oil and lemon juice in a food processor and pureeing until smooth.

Blanch the beans in boiling water for 4 minutes. Drain and refresh in cold water. From a cold water start, boil the eggs for three minutes. Refresh in cold water, peel and cut into quarters.

Heavily coat the tuna fillets with the pepper and a pinch of salt.

Heat a frying pan, add the oil, and over a high heat cook the tuna for 2 minutes each side, or to your liking.

In a bowl, gently toss the beans, eggs, spinach and olives together and drizzle with the dressing. Divide equally on two plates, top with the tuna and serve.

Note: You can substitute tinned tuna.

SALMON AND SILVERBEET PIE

Serves 4

500ml (16fl oz) cream
1 teaspoon nutmeg powder
Grated zest of 1 lemon
1 bunch silverbeet, washed and stalks
removed
400g (13oz) poached salmon, flaked
Olive oil spray

1 bunch basil, washed, leaves picked and
chopped
2 sheets puff pastry, 30cmx30cm
(12insx12ins)
1 egg, lightly beaten
1 tablespoon fennel seeds

Pre-heat oven to moderate, 180°C (350°F) Gas Mark 4.

Simmer the cream, nutmeg and lemon zest on a low heat for 10 minutes. Blanch the silverbeet for three minutes in a pot of boiling water. Drain and refresh in cold water. Place in a tea towel and ring out excess water.

Flake the salmon by gently pulling apart into bite-size pieces. Place in a large bowl with the silverbeet, basil and cream and mix together until combined.

Spray a 30 x 3cm (12 x 1¼ins) deep fluted flan tin with olive oil and line the base with 1 sheet of puff pastry. Spoon the silverbeet and salmon on to the pastry and smooth out evenly. Place the remaining sheet of puff pastry on top, allowing it to overhang the flan tin. Press the edges of the pastry with your fingers to seal the pie. Trim off any excess pastry with a small sharp knife and then brush the top of the pastry with the egg and sprinkle with fennel seeds. Bake for 40 minutes.

Note: Tinned salmon can be substituted. For a healthier option use reduced-fat cream.

CANADIAN PLANK SALMON

Serves 6

My Canadian sous chef, Eric Bradley, shared this recipe with me when we worked together at Parliament House in Sydney. The presentation is impressive and the flavour is amazing as the fish has a slight smoky taste (see picture pages 96 and 97).

50cm x 30cm (20ins x 12ins) cedar wood plank, untreated
1 side salmon, pin bones removed (ask your fishmonger)
1 bunch thyme, stalks removed and leaves chopped
Juice of 1 lemon
¼ cup (60ml/2fl oz) Dijon mustard
¼ cup (60ml/2fl oz) olive oil
1 cup rock salt

Submerge the cedar wood in water and soak overnight.
Marinate the salmon in Dijon mustard, thyme and lemon juice for at least 1 hour but preferably 2. Pre-heat the barbecue (grill) to a medium heat and place the cedar plank on the barbecue griddle.
Sprinkle rock salt on the top of the plank and close the barbecue lid for 10 minutes or until the salt starts to pop. Place the salmon skin side down on rock salt. Close the barbecue lid and cook on a medium heat for 25 minutes, or to your liking.
The salmon presents beautifully as a centrepiece on the dining table. Be sure to place heatproof mats on your dining table before placing the cedar plank on it.

Note: Cedar wood can be purchased from a timber yard. Make sure you specify untreated wood. If the plank catches fire put it out using a water spray.

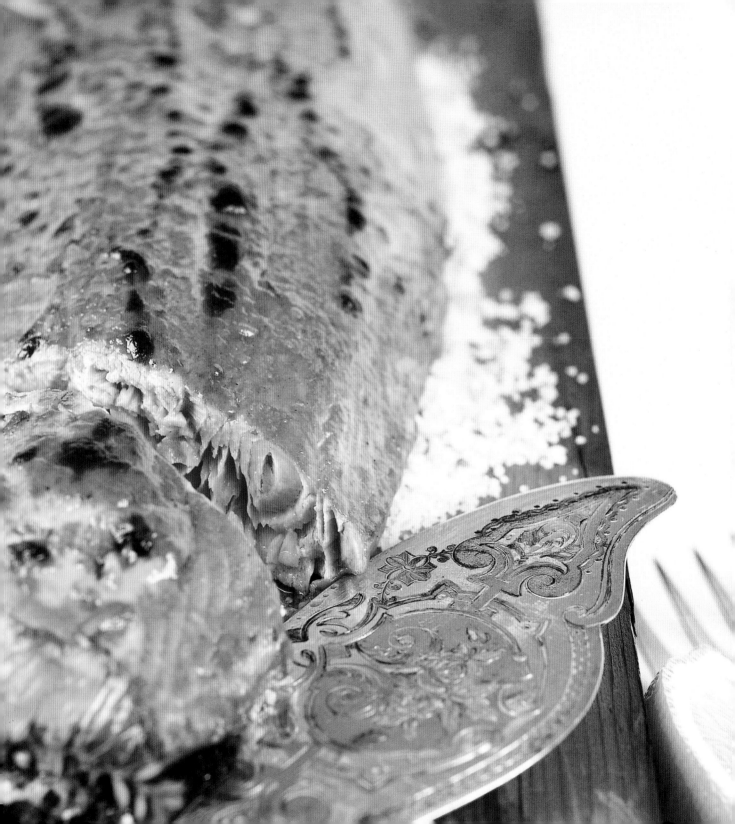

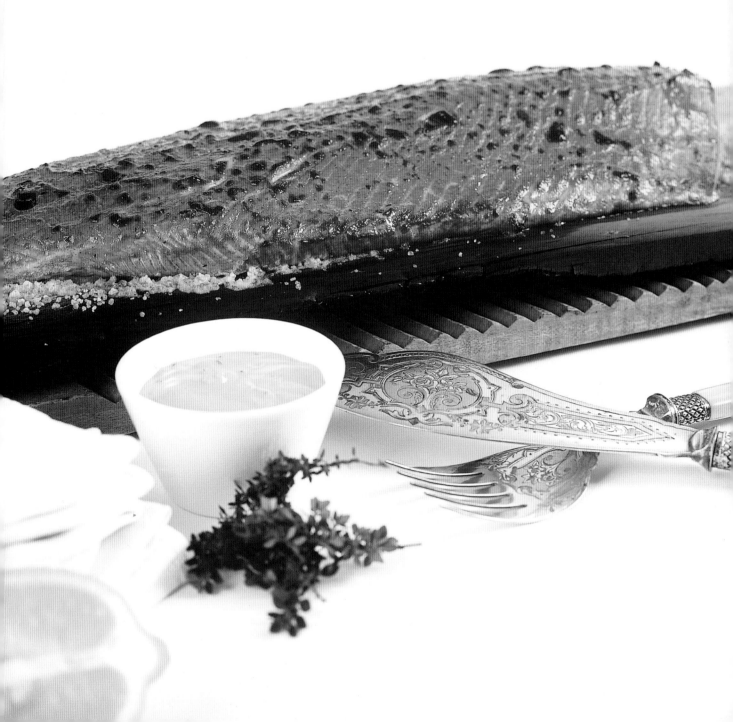

Canadian Plank Salmon

PEPPERED RARE TROUT ON ASIAN GREENS WITH SAKE AND MIRIN DRESSING

Serves 2

1 tablespoon Cajun spice powder

1 tablespoon cayenne pepper

½ cup plain flour

2 tablespoons light olive oil

2 x 200g (6½oz) trout fillets

1 bunch baby bok choy (pak choi),
washed and cut in quarters

100g (3½oz) pickled ginger

Combine the Cajun spice, cayenne pepper and flour and coat the trout fillets with the spice mix.

Heat the olive oil in a large pan and cook the trout for 3 minutes on each side, or to your liking.

Blanch the bok choy for 4 minutes in a pot of boiling water. Drain and equally divide on two plates. Place trout on top, drizzle with the dressing and sprinkle with pickled ginger (see picture page 100).

Dressing

1 cup (250ml/8fl oz) sake
½ cup mirin
2 tablespoons soy sauce
2 tablespoons cornflour
2 tablespoons water

Bring the sake, mirin, and soy sauce to the boil. Mix the cornflour and water to make a paste, then add to the sauce and stir until thickened. Keep warm until needed.

Note: Mirin is a sweet rice-based wine used in Japanese cuisine. There are two types: hon mirin which contains about 14% alcohol and shin mirin, which has less than 1% alcohol. The flavour of both is the same. I use hon mirin but if you prefer less alcohol substitute shin mirin. Both are available at Asian grocers and the Asian sections of large supermarkets.

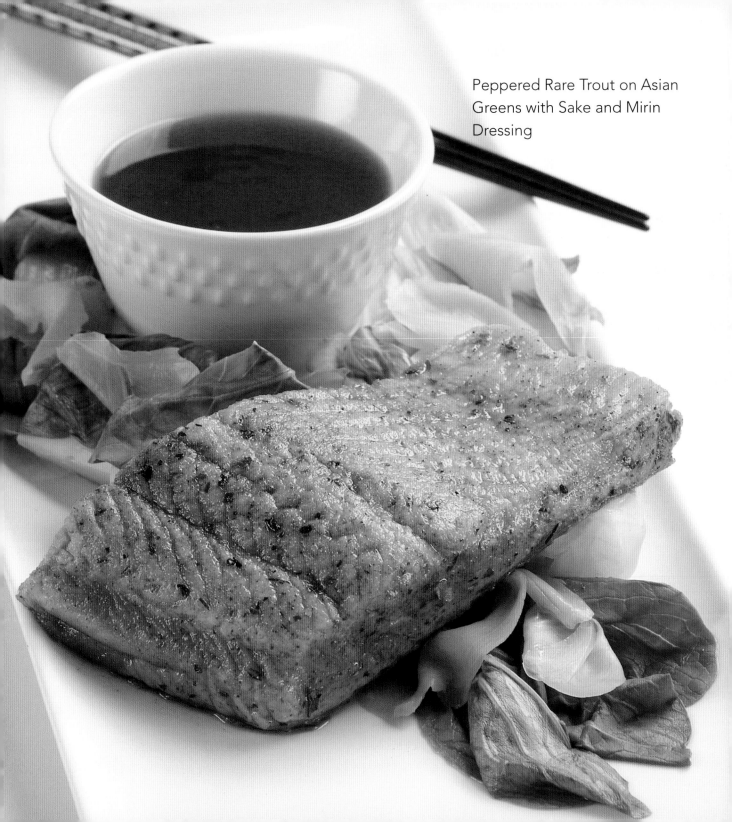

Peppered Rare Trout on Asian Greens with Sake and Mirin Dressing

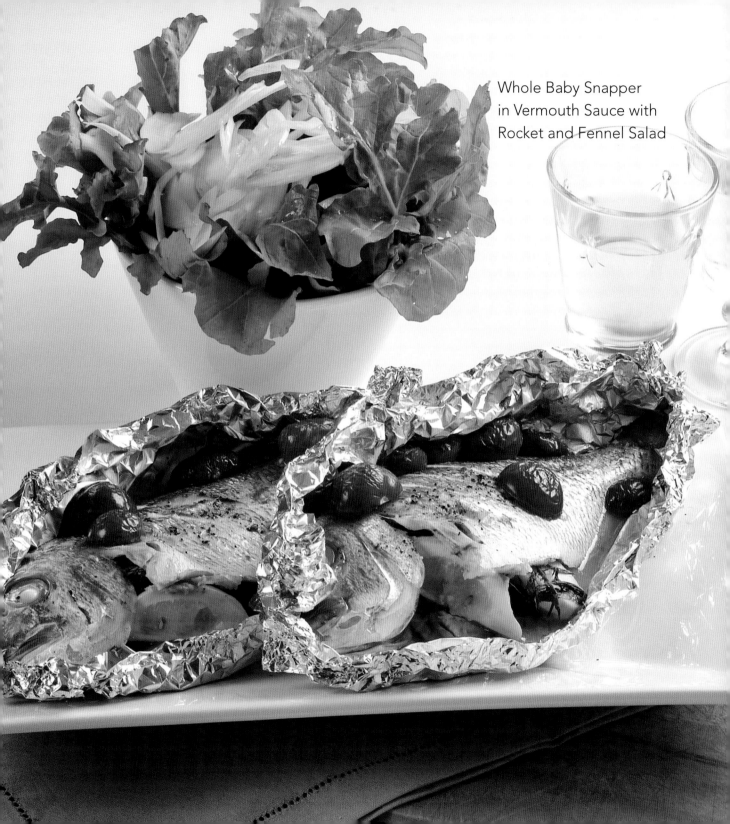

Whole Baby Snapper
in Vermouth Sauce with
Rocket and Fennel Salad

WHOLE BABY SNAPPER IN VERMOUTH SAUCE WITH ROCKET AND FENNEL SALAD

Serves 2

2 whole baby snapper,
  400–420g
  (13–14oz) each
1 lemon, quartered
8 sprigs dill
2 fresh bay leaves
Sea salt

100g (3½ oz) butter, diced
100ml (3fl oz) vermouth
200ml (6fl oz) white wine
1 bunch rocket, washed
  and stalks trimmed
1 baby fennel bulb, washed
  and finely shaved

½ punnet cherry
  tomatoes, washed and
  cut in halves
2 tablespoons extra virgin
  olive oil

Pre-heat oven to moderate, 180°C (350°F) Gas Mark 4.

Score the fish three times on each side by cutting about 1cm (½ in) deep in to the skin and flesh. Stuff each fish cavity with 2 lemon quarters, 4 dill sprigs and 1 bay leaf. Sprinkle each fish with sea salt and wrap separately in a 30cm (12ins) piece of foil. Bring the sides of the foil up around the fish and crimp ends together tightly, leaving the top open.

Put equal quantities of the diced butter and cherry tomatoes on top of each fish, pour over equal amounts of vermouth and white wine and then seal parcels.

Cook for 15–20 minutes. Place the fish on warmed plates and allow each person to open their parcel. Toss the rocket leaves and fennel together with the extra virgin olive oil. Sprinkle to taste with salt and serve (see picture page 101).

Note: You should be able to get fresh bay leaves at your greengrocer. If they are unavailable substitute dried bay leaves.

BAKED TROUT STUFFED WITH SPINACH AND PINE NUTS

Serves 2

1 bunch English spinach, washed and
   roots trimmed
1 small bulb fennel, washed, tops
   removed and finely sliced
100g (3½oz) pine nuts, dry roasted

Grated zest of 1 lemon
2 plate-sized trout, 400g (13oz) each,
   gutted and scaled
Sea salt and freshly ground black pepper
2 tablespoons olive oil

Pre-heat oven to moderate, 180°C (350°F) Gas Mark 4.
Blanch the spinach for two minutes in boiling water. Drain and refresh in cold water.
Mix together the spinach, fennel, pine nuts, lemon zest, a pinch of salt and pepper
and fill the trout cavity until plump. Rub each fish with oil and a little salt. Place the
trout on a baking tray lined with baking paper and cook for 15 minutes.
Serve immediately.

SEARED TUNA WITH GREEN MANGO SALAD

Serves 2

Green Mango Salad
50g (2oz) snow peas
 (mange tout/
sugar peas), strung and
 finely sliced
1 green mango, peeled
 and finely sliced
1 cup bean sprouts
½ bunch mint, leaves
 washed and picked

2 tablespoons unsalted
 peanuts, crushed

Salad Dressing
2 tablespoons sesame oil
1 tablespoon fish sauce
2 tablespoons lime juice
1 bird's-eye chilli, seeds
 removed and finely
 chopped

2 tablespoons white
 sesame seeds
2 tablespoons black
 sesame seeds
Sea salt
2 x 200g (6½ oz) yellow fin
 tuna steaks
1 tablespoon light olive oil

Toss all the salad ingredients together. Combine the salad dressing ingredients in a small jug. Place the sesame seeds and a pinch of salt on a plate.
Roll the tuna steaks in the mixture until well coated. You will find the seeds will stick easily to the moist fish.
Heat the oil in a frying pan and cook the tuna over a high heat for 2 minutes each side, or to your liking.
Divide the salad on two plates, top with the tuna, drizzle with the dressing and serve.

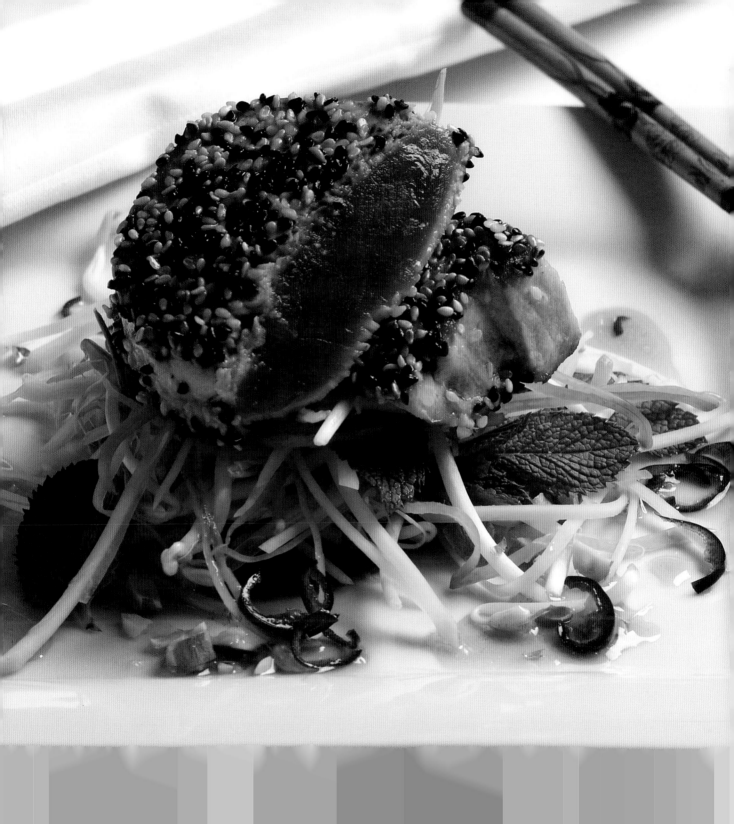

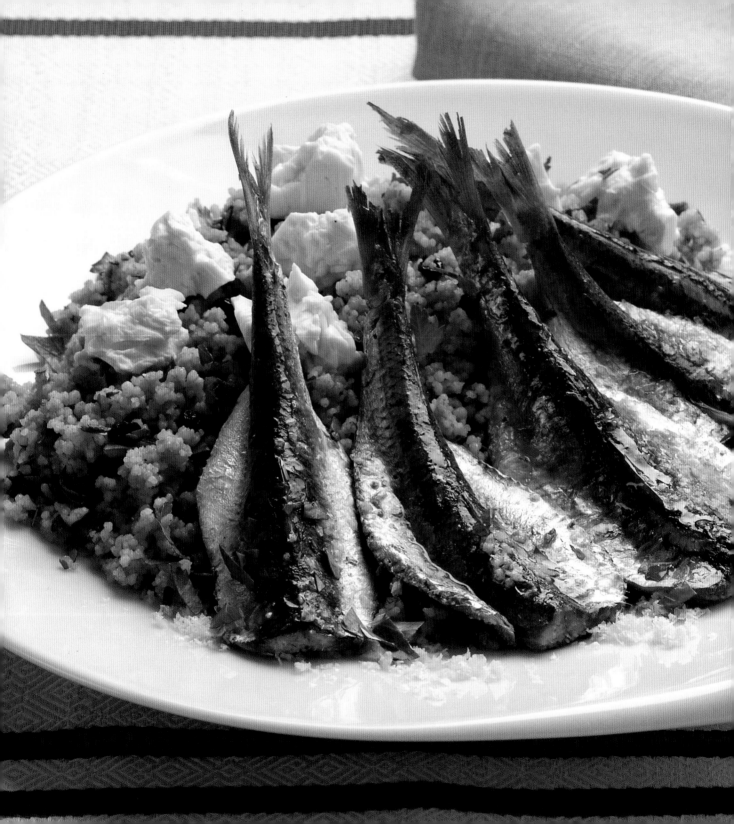

GRILLED SARDINES ON COUSCOUS SALAD

Serves 2

1 cup couscous
2 cups (500ml/16fl oz) orange juice
1 teaspoon cinnamon
2 tablespoons currants
1 bunch parsley, washed, leaves picked and roughly chopped

12 fresh sardine fillets
2 tablespoons light olive oil
Sea salt, to taste
150g (2oz) low-fat feta, crumbled
¼ cup (60ml/2fl oz) extra virgin olive oil

Put the couscous in a small bowl. In a pan, bring the orange juice, cinnamon and currants to the boil and pour over the couscous. Cover the bowl with cling wrap and leave for 5 minutes. Fluff the couscous with a fork and toss together with half the parsley leaves.

Coat the sardine fillets with olive oil and sprinkle with sea salt. Grill (broil) on a medium heat, flesh side up, for 5 minutes.

Spoon the couscous mixture on two plates and top with the sardines. Sprinkle with the feta and remaining parsley. Drizzle with the extra virgin olive oil and serve.

Note: Ask your fishmonger for sardine fillets. The head and all bones will be removed. Tinned sardines can be substituted. Drain a 200g (6½oz) tin of sardines, place the sardines on a flat tray and put under the grill for 3 minutes or until just slightly warmed.

WHOLE POACHED SALMON

Many a cook is hesitant to try poaching a whole salmon but it really isn't such a difficult thing to do and when served with chat potatoes, asparagus and English spinach with dill and mint mayonnaise, it is an incredible show-stopper. A whole salmon tastes sensational too and looks so special when you serve it. You'll also find that a poached salmon goes a long way. Start with the whole fish and then use what's left over to create four other delicious meals.

Dill and Mint Mayonnaise
¼ cup (60ml/2fl oz) whole egg mayonnaise (see recipe page 110)
½ bunch mint, washed and finely chopped
½ bunch dill, washed and finely chopped
Freshly ground black pepper

Poaching Liquid
2 litres (3½ pints) water
750ml (24fl oz) dry white wine
500ml (16fl oz) white wine vinegar
2 bay leaves, dried
½ bunch of celery, washed and roughly chopped
1 teaspoon black peppercorns

1 whole salmon (1.5–1.75kg/3–3½lbs), gutted and scaled
200g (6½oz) chat potatoes, cut in halves
1 bunch asparagus
1 bunch English spinach, washed and dried

Combine the mayonnaise ingredients in a small bowl and set aside.

Bring the poaching liquid ingredients to the boil for 5 minutes. Place the salmon in the fish kettle and cover with the boiled liquid until it is submerged. Simmer for 18–20 minutes.

Peel the potatoes and from a cold water start boil for 7 minutes or until tender.

Blanch the asparagus in salted boiling water for 4 minutes and lightly blanch the spinach for 2 minutes.

Remove the salmon from the fish kettle, allowing the excess water to drain away. Make an incision along the backbone from the end of the tail to the back of head behind the gills, then gently cut the skin straight across the base of the tail. Gently peel off the skin. Turn the salmon over and repeat the process.

Gently place on a warm platter, put the vegetables on another platter and serve. Serve the dill and mint mayonnaise separately.

Note: A fish kettle is ideal for poaching salmon because it comes with an internal rack on which you place the fish while it is cooking. It allows you to remove the salmon easily without damaging its flesh. If you don't have one use a deep baking dish and cover with foil while poaching and carefully turn the salmon every 10 minutes. Store-bought mayonnaise can be substituted but it will not have as good a flavour as homemade mayonnaise. For a healthier option use low-fat mayonnaise.

HOMEMADE MAYONNAISE

2 egg yolks, room temperature
1 teaspoon Dijon mustard
300ml (10fl oz) light olive oil
1 tablespoon white wine vinegar
Sea salt and freshly ground black pepper

Place the egg yolks and mustard in a food processor.
On a low speed slowly add half the olive oil until mixture becomes thick and creamy.
Add vinegar and continue to add the remainder of the oil. Season to taste with salt and pepper.

Note: Mayonnaise can be stored in a refrigerator for up to a week.

POACHED SALMON AND LINGUINE WITH CHERRY TOMATOES, GARLIC AND ROCKET

Serves 2

200g (6½oz) poached salmon, flaked
200g (6½oz) linguine
¼ cup (60ml/2fl oz) light olive oil
3 cloves garlic, sliced

½ punnet cherry tomatoes, washed
100g (3½oz) wild rocket, washed and
  dried
Sea salt and freshly ground black pepper

Flake the salmon by gently pulling apart into bite-size pieces.

Bring a large pot of salted water to the boil, add the linguine and boil for 15 minutes or until al dente.

Heat the olive oil in a large frying pan, add the garlic and cook for 3 minutes. Add the cherry tomatoes and salmon and cook for a further 2 minutes.

Gently toss through the linguine, add the rocket, season to taste with salt and pepper and serve.

Note: Tinned salmon can be substituted. Wild rocket does not need to be chopped or torn as the leaves are quite small. The rocket will slightly wilt once tossed through the linguine.

POACHED SALMON WITH GRILLED ASPARAGUS AND POACHED EGGS

Serves 2

4 spears asparagus, woody stalks
   trimmed
Olive oil
Sea salt and freshly ground black pepper
200g (6½oz) poached salmon, flaked

2 soft poached eggs
25g (1oz) parmesan cheese, shaved
½ bunch chervil, leaves washed, picked
   and chopped

Pre-heat oven to moderate, 180°C (350°F) Gas Mark 4.
Lightly blanch the asparagus for 4 minutes. Drain and refresh in cold water.
Pre-heat the griddle plate until smoking. Coat the asparagus in olive oil, a little salt and pepper and cook on griddle plate for 5 minutes. Place the salmon on a tray and reheat in the oven for 5 minutes or until warmed through.
Arrange the asparagus on warmed plates and top with the salmon. Place the poached egg beside the salmon. Sprinkle the shaved parmesan over the egg, then sprinkle the chopped chervil over the entire dish and serve.

Note: Use a vegetable peeler to shave the cheese. Chervil is not available all year round especially in the warmer months; parsley is a perfect substitute.

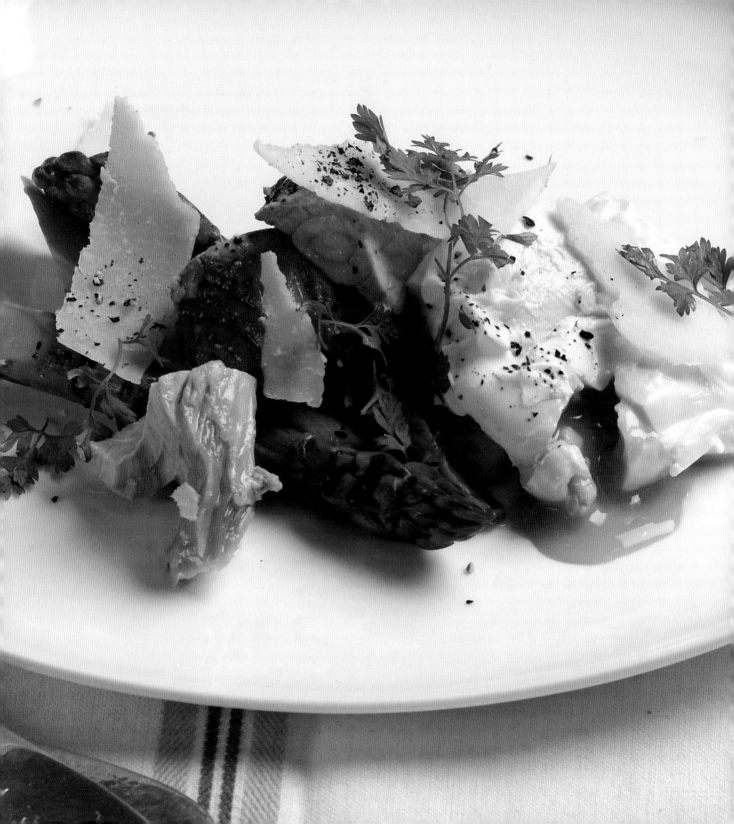

HOW TO PERFECTLY POACH AN EGG

- Bring a small saucepan of water and 1 tablespoon of white vinegar to the simmer. Crack an egg into a bowl and gently slide it into simmering water. Allow to cook for three minutes and remove with a slotted spoon.

- Note: Poached eggs need to be quite soft when serving with fish and vegetables. When poaching eggs to serve on toast for breakfast, cook them for at least 5 minutes or to your liking.

WATERCRESS AND PEACH SALAD TOSSED WITH POACHED SALMON

Serves 2

200g (6½oz) poached salmon, flaked
1 bunch watercress, leaves picked,
  washed and dried
1 ripe peach, skin on, sliced

100ml (3fl oz) verjuice
100ml (3fl oz) extra virgin olive oil
Sea salt and freshly ground black pepper

Flake the salmon by gently pulling apart into bite-sized pieces. Toss the watercress leaves with the sliced peach, add the salmon.
Make the dressing by combining the verjuice and the extra virgin olive oil in a small bowl.
Season to taste with salt and pepper and drizzle over the salad.

Note: If peaches are out of season paw paw makes an excellent substitute.

POACHED SALMON AND LEMON RISOTTO

Serves 2

200g (6½oz) poached salmon, flaked
1 tablespoon light virgin olive oil
25g (1oz) butter
1 white onion, finely diced
Sea salt
300g (9½oz) Arborio rice

Grated zest and juice of 1 lemon
600ml (1 pint) fish stock
2 tablespoons fresh parmesan cheese, grated
½ bunch flat leaf parsley, washed and chopped

Flake the salmon by gently pulling apart into bite-sized pieces.
Heat a large heavy-based saucepan and then add the oil, half the butter, the onion and salt to taste. Cook over a low heat until the onion is soft but not brown.
Add the rice and stir for a few minutes to ensure all the grains are coated. Increase heat to high, add the lemon zest and juice.
Heat the fish stock in a separate saucepan and gradually add to the rice, stirring continuously until all the liquid is absorbed.
Add salmon and remainder of butter until melted and salmon is warmed through.
The risotto should be quite wet and slightly runny.
Sprinkle with parmesan and parsley and serve.

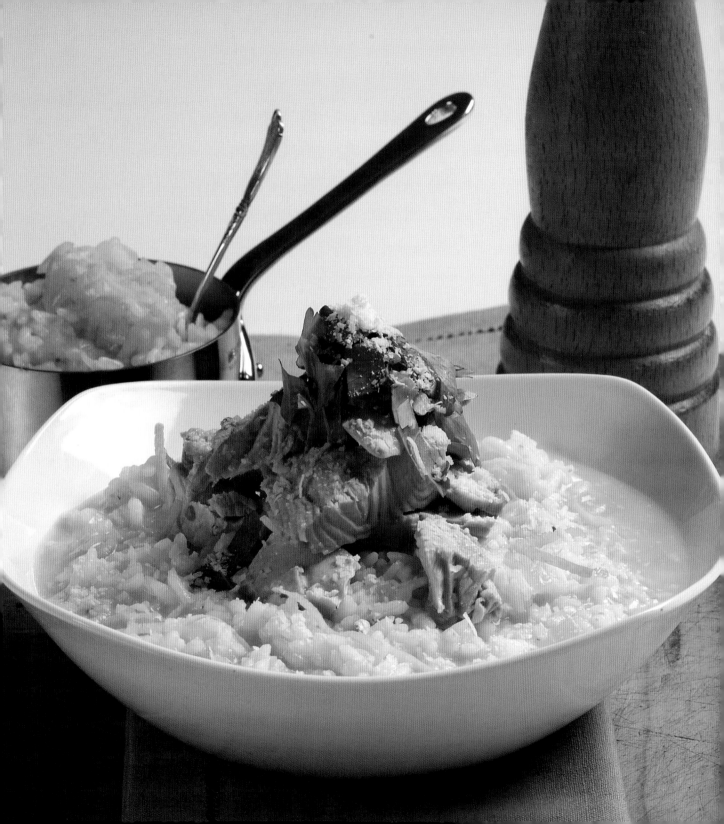

QUICK WAYS WITH OYSTERS

- Mix 150ml (5fl oz) tomato juice, 3 drops Tabasco and ½ teaspoon smoked paprika powder together. Pour over fresh or bottled oysters in chilled cocktail glasses. Add a cucumber swizzle stick.

- Serve tinned smoked oysters on Melba toast topped with a sprinkle of cayenne pepper.

Serve fresh oysters in their shells with:

- A splash of champagne over each one: French is wicked but oh so nice!

- Salsa: mix together chopped mint leaves, diced mango and a little finely sliced chilli. Spoon over the oysters.

- A touch of spice: put a small dollop of tomato chilli jam on each oyster.

QUICK WAYS WITH TINNED SARDINES

Drain a 110g (3½ oz) tin of sardines and serve:
- As a dip: mash sardines with tahini, a little reduced-fat sour cream, lemon juice and chopped parsley.

- For lunch: mash and mix with finely chopped onion and lemon juice. Spread slices of toasted sourdough bread with hummus and cover with sardines.

- As a salad: toss with 1 cup of cannellini beans, ½ a finely chopped capsicum (sweet pepper/bell pepper), 1 finely sliced garlic clove and 1 diced apple. Pile on lettuce. Add a squeeze of lemon, a splash of extra virgin olive oil and some chopped parsley.

- For dinner: mix sardines with a tin of chopped tomatoes, 1 finely sliced chilli, ½ cup pine nuts and stir through fusilli pasta. Sprinkle with chopped basil leaves.

QUICK WAYS WITH TINNED TUNA

Drain a 225g (7 oz) tin of tuna and:
- Toss in a bowl with a squeeze of lemon juice, bean shoots and parsley leaves. Serve in a crisp iceberg lettuce leaf.

- Toss with diced red capsicum (sweet pepper/bell pepper) and Spanish onion. Coat with a little mayonnaise. Cut a round bread roll in half and put a few baby spinach leaves with tuna on top of one half of the bread roll. Place the other half on top. Grill (broil) in a sandwich maker.

- Blanch some green beans, refresh in iced water, and toss with kalamata and Sardinia olives. Top with tinned tuna, a little chopped parsley, and extra virgin olive oil.

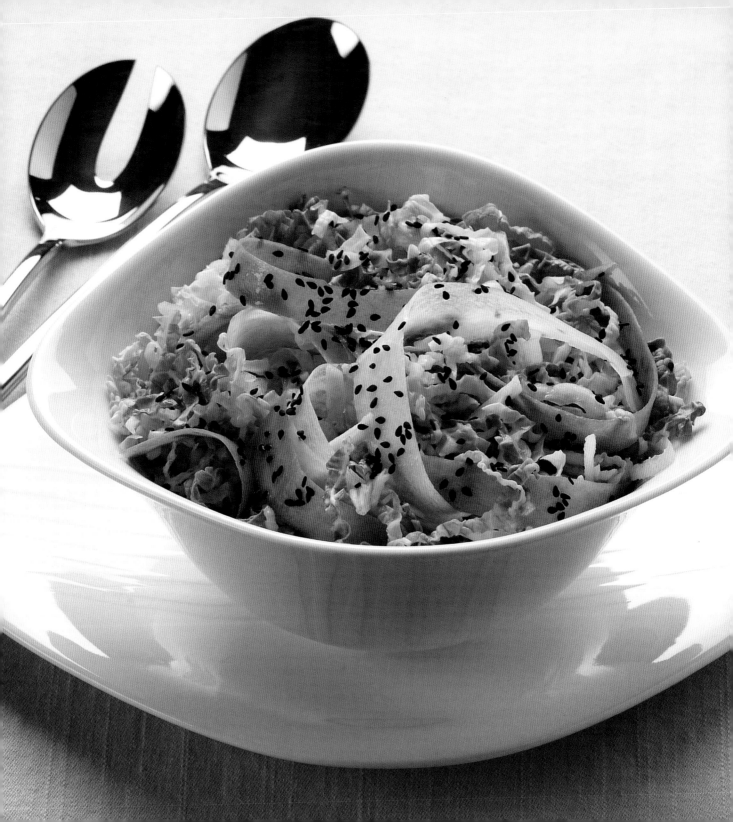

Five

THE VEGGIE PATCH

Vegetables are often taken for granted, overcooked, and served without much thought but they deserve better. I consider them a culinary challenge as well as a delight.

When I'm creating a new dish with vegetables I spend a great deal of time thinking about how the flavours and aromas will work best together. For instance, mixing peas with zucchinis in Pea, Zucchini, Mint and Potato Salad with Seeded Mustard Dressing complements all the flavours without being overpowering.

For optimum eye health you should eat plenty of vegetables and fresh fruit daily because your eyes need plenty of Vitamins C and E. Vitamin C is found in broccoli, potatoes, capsicums (sweet pepper/bell pepper), tomatoes and citrus fruit, while Vitamin E is found in green leafy vegetables such as spinach and broccoli as well as asparagus, capsicum and avocado. Papaya and peaches also contain Vitamin E.

Dark green leafy vegetables, particularly all varieties of spinach, are high in lutein, an important antioxidant for eye health.

Vegetables should be cooked quickly and for the shortest possible amount of time so that they always look their best when served. Overcooking makes them soggy and colourless.

There's really nothing you can't do with vegetables. They can be served as an appetiser, as an accompaniment to meat or fish, or as a complete meal on their own. You can serve them raw as well as cooked and with or without sauces. Vegetable cuisine is in a class all of its own.

JAPANESE COLESLAW

Dressing
¼ cup (60ml/2fl oz) mirin
1 tablespoon sesame oil
Juice of 2 lemons
1 tablespoon Japanese rice vinegar
1 clove garlic, minced

½ wombok cabbage (Chinese cabbage),
   washed and shredded
1 carrot, peeled and grated
1 daikon (white radish), peeled and
   grated
2 Fuji apples, peeled and grated
1 tablespoon black sesame seeds

Make the dressing by whisking together all the ingredients in a bowl until combined. Toss the cabbage, carrot, daikon and apple together in a serving bowl. Pour over the dressing, sprinkle with sesame seeds (see picture page 120).

Note: Mirin is a sweet rice-based wine used in Japanese cuisine. There are two types: hon mirin which contains about 14% alcohol and shin mirin, which has less than 1% alcohol. The flavour of both is the same. I use hon mirin. If you prefer less alcohol substitute shin mirin. Both are available at Asian grocers and the Asian sections of large supermarkets.

FIELD MUSHROOMS WITH GREMOLATA

Serves 2

1 large bunch parsley, washed and leaves
   picked
2 cloves garlic
Grated zest of 1 lemon
150ml (5fl oz) extra virgin olive oil

Sea salt and freshly ground black pepper
100ml (3fl oz) light olive oil
500g (1lb) field mushrooms, peeled and
   stalks trimmed

To make the gremolata, put the parsley, garlic, lemon zest and extra virgin olive oil in a food processor and blend to make a paste. Add a pinch of salt and pepper and put to one side.

Heat a large frying pan to medium-low heat, add the oil and gently cook mushrooms for 8 minutes or until soft.

Serve in warm bowls and sprinkle with the gremolata.

ROAST GOLDEN NUGGET PUMPKIN FILLED WITH INDIAN SPICED VEGETABLES

Serves 4

This makes a wonderful starter or a light meal.

4 small golden nugget pumpkins
¼ cup (60ml/2fl oz) olive oil
¼ cup chat masala spice mix
1 medium potato, diced
4 baby eggplants (aubergines), diced
4 baby carrots, peeled and tops trimmed

½ cup tinned corn kernels, drained
150ml (5fl oz) water
200ml (6fl oz) lite coconut cream
1 bunch broccolini, washed and woody
   ends trimmed
cream sauce and serve immediately.

Pre-heat oven to moderate, 180°C (350°F) Gas Mark 4.
Slice the tops off the pumpkins, scoop out the seeds and discard. Place on a flat baking tray, dribble the olive oil over the pumpkins and cook for 20–25 minutes.
In a saucepan, gently dry roast the chat masala spice mix on a low heat for 3 minutes or until aromatic, occasionally stirring to prevent it from burning. Add the potato, eggplant, carrots and corn and sauté for a further 5 minutes then add the water and coconut cream and simmer for 20 minutes. Add in the broccolini and simmer for a further 8 minutes. Fill the pumpkins with the vegetables, pour over the coconut

Note: Broccoli can be substituted for broccolini.

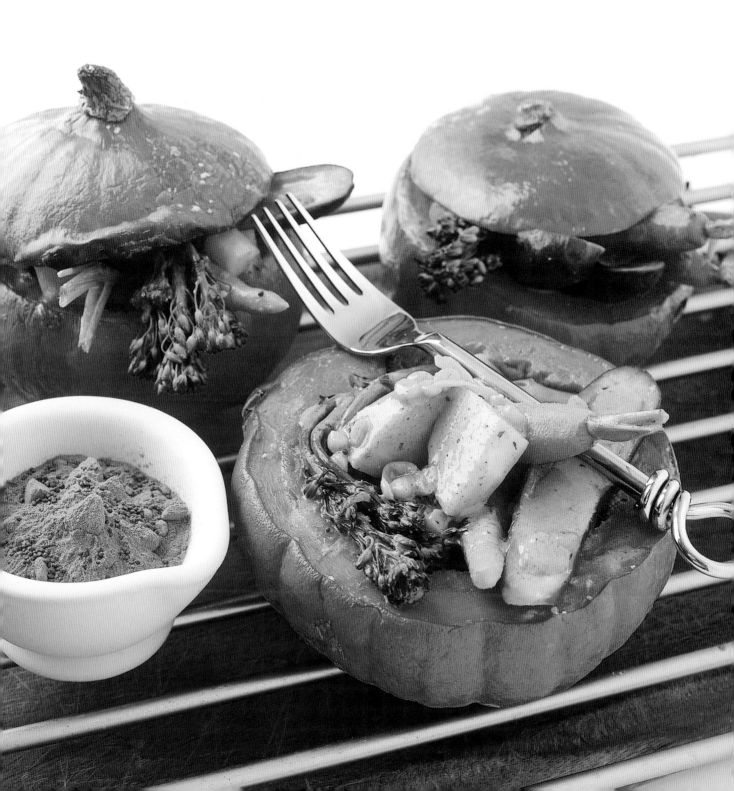

ZUCCHINI AND BASIL FRITTERS WITH CRÈME FRAÎCHE

Makes 8 fritters

Serve topped with poached salmon if it takes your fancy!

1 tablespoon unsalted butter
3 large zucchinis (courgettes), washed
  and grated
2 tablespoons basil, washed and
  chopped
3 green shallots (spring onions/scallions),
washed and chopped
2 eggs, lightly beaten
½ cup Japanese breadcrumbs
Sea salt and freshly ground black pepper
2 tablespoons light olive oil
200g (6½oz) crème fraîche

Heat the butter in a frying pan and sauté the zucchini, basil and shallots for 3 minutes. Place in a bowl and allow to cool, then drain off any excess liquid. Add the eggs, breadcrumbs and salt and pepper to taste.

Heat a frying pan with the olive oil to a medium heat and cook heaped tablespoons of zucchini mix for 3 minutes on each side or until golden brown. Remove and rest on absorbent paper towel. Top each fritter with a dollop of crème fraîche and serve warm.

Note: Japanese breadcrumbs are slightly coarser than regular breadcrumbs and are available at Asian grocers and the Asian sections of large supermarkets. For a healthier option substitute reduced-fat sour cream for the crème fraîche.

TURMERIC SPICED POTATOES

4 sebago potatoes
Sea salt
2 tablespoons olive oil
1 tablespoon black mustard seeds
2 curry leaves
1 teaspoon chilli powder

1 tablespoon turmeric powder
1 tablespoon coriander (cilantro) powder
1 tablespoon cumin powder
1 teaspoon sugar
250ml (8fl oz) water
1 bunch mint, washed and chopped

Peel the potatoes and cut into 5cm (2ins) cubes. Cook in a pan of salted boiling water for 4 minutes, drain and set aside.

Heat the olive oil in a frying pan, add the black mustard seeds and stir well until fragrant and starting to pop. Add the curry leaves and stir. Continue to stir while adding the chilli, turmeric, coriander, cumin, a pinch of salt and sugar. Cook for 1 minute, stirring all the time.

Add the water and potatoes and simmer for 5 minutes or until potatoes are cooked. Sprinkle with the mint.

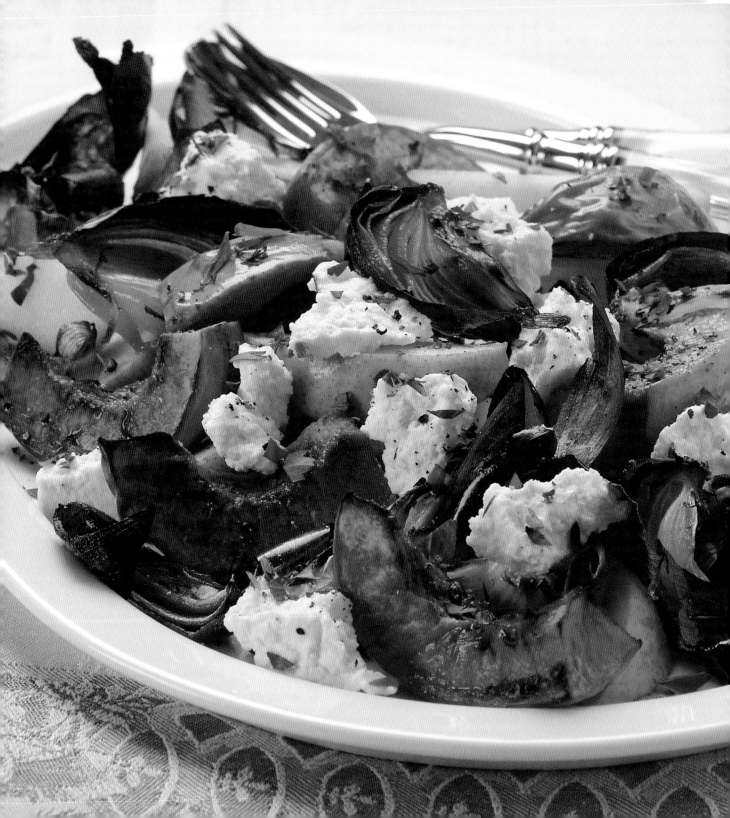

SLOW ROASTED VEGETABLE SALAD WITH PEARS AND RICOTTA

Serves 4 as a side dish

1 butternut pumpkin, skin on, deseeded
2 Spanish onions, not peeled
¼ cup (60ml/2fl oz) olive oil
Sea salt and freshly ground black pepper

3 dessert pears
250g (2oz) low-fat fresh ricotta
½ bunch flat leaf parsley, leaves washed
  and picked, roughly chopped

Pre-heat oven to moderately slow, 160°C (325°F) Gas Mark 3.
Cut the pumpkin and onions into wedges, drizzle with the olive oil and sprinkle with
a little salt and pepper and bake for 30 minutes. Arrange the warm pumpkin and
onions on a platter, cut the pears into quarters and scatter over the top.
Crumble over the ricotta, sprinkle with parsley and serve.

BRAISED PUY LENTILS WITH CARAMELISED ROOT VEGETABLES AND MINTED YOGHURT

Serves 4

1 sweet potato, peeled and cut into wedges

2 parsnips, peeled and cut into wedges

1 swede, peeled and cut into wedges

2 tablespoons olive oil

Sea salt

1 brown onion, diced

2 cloves garlic, crushed

2 cups puy lentils

2 cups (500ml/16fl oz) reduced-salt packet beef stock

1 cup (250ml/8fl oz) red wine

1/3 cup (80ml/2½ fl oz) low-fat natural yoghurt

1 teaspoon cumin powder

1 tablespoon honey

1 bunch mint, washed and chopped

Pre-heat oven to moderate, 180°C (350°F) Gas Mark 4. Gently roll the sweet potato, parsnip and swede in 1 tablespoon of olive oil. Sprinkle with a little salt and bake for 30 minutes or until tender.

Heat the remaining oil in a medium saucepan and sauté the onions and garlic. Add the lentils, stock and red wine and simmer for 30 minutes or until tender.

To make the minted yoghurt, mix the yoghurt, cumin, honey and mint until well combined. Serve the lentils topped with roasted vegetables, a dollop of minted yoghurt and a sprinkle of extra chopped mint.

Note: Puy lentils are small French green lentils, sometimes described as blue lentils. Green lentils can be substituted in this recipe.

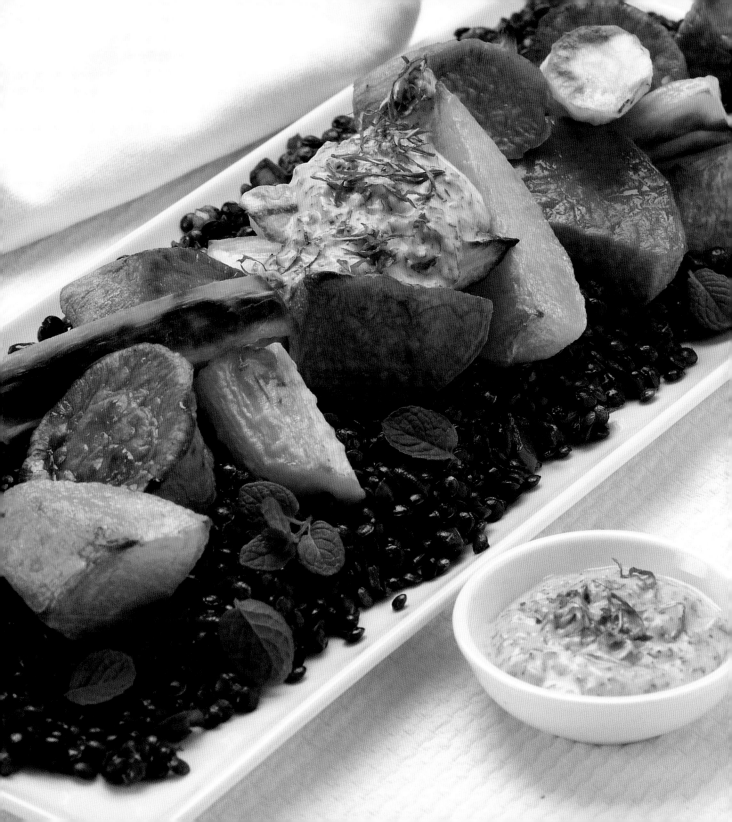

PEA, ZUCCHINI, MINT AND POTATO SALAD WITH SEEDED MUSTARD DRESSING

Serves 2

3 zucchinis (courgettes), washed and diced

300g (9½oz) waxy potatoes, washed

¼ cup (60ml/2fl oz) homemade mayonnaise (See Chapter Four, From the Ocean)

1 tablespoon seeded mustard

1 tablespoon extra virgin olive oil

1 bunch mint, washed, leaves picked and chopped

1 cup frozen baby peas, defrosted

Blanch the zucchinis in boiling water for 4 minutes. Drain and refresh in cold water. From a cold water start, boil the potatoes for 5 minutes or until tender, refresh with cold water, peel and slice. Combine the mayonnaise, mustard and the extra virgin olive oil. Place the zucchinis, potatoes, mint, peas and mayonnaise dressing in a serving bowl and mix until lightly coated.

Note: Store-bought mayonnaise can be substituted but it will not have as good a flavour as homemade mayonnaise. For a healthier option use low-fat mayonnaise.

WINTER VEGETABLE AND PEARL BARLEY SOUP

Serves 6

2 tablespoons light olive oil

3 cloves garlic, crushed

1 large onion, diced

1 cup pearl barley

1 cup (250ml/8fl oz) white wine

3 litres (5¼ pints) chicken stock

2 medium potatoes, diced

2 parsnips, peeled and diced

3 large carrots, peeled and diced

3 zucchinis (courgettes), washed and diced

4 plump ripe tomatoes, washed and diced

3 celery sticks, washed and diced

Sea salt and freshly ground black pepper

1 small bunch flat leaf parsley, washed and chopped

Heat the olive oil in a large heavy-based pot and sauté the garlic and onion. Add the barley, wine and stock, bring to the boil and simmer for 30 minutes. Stir in the potatoes, parsnips and carrots and simmer for another 10 minutes.

Add the zucchinis, tomatoes and celery and simmer for a further 7 minutes. Season to taste with salt and pepper.

Sprinkle with freshly chopped parsley and serve immediately.

PICKLED CARROTS WITH POPPY SEEDS

Serves 4 as a side dish

Toss the carrots through a garden salad and serve with grilled (broiled) fish and spinach, or serve as a side dish with your favourite Indian curry.

2 cups (500ml/16fl oz) white wine vinegar
¾ cup white sugar
1 bay leaf, dried

2 large carrots, peeled and julienned
2 tablespoons poppy seeds

Simmer the vinegar, sugar and bay leaf together in a small saucepan for 5 minutes or until sugar has dissolved.
Remove from the heat and stir in the carrots and poppy seeds.
Spoon carrots and liquid into a sterilised jar and seal.

Note: The carrots can be stored for a month in the pantry or refrigerated for two months.

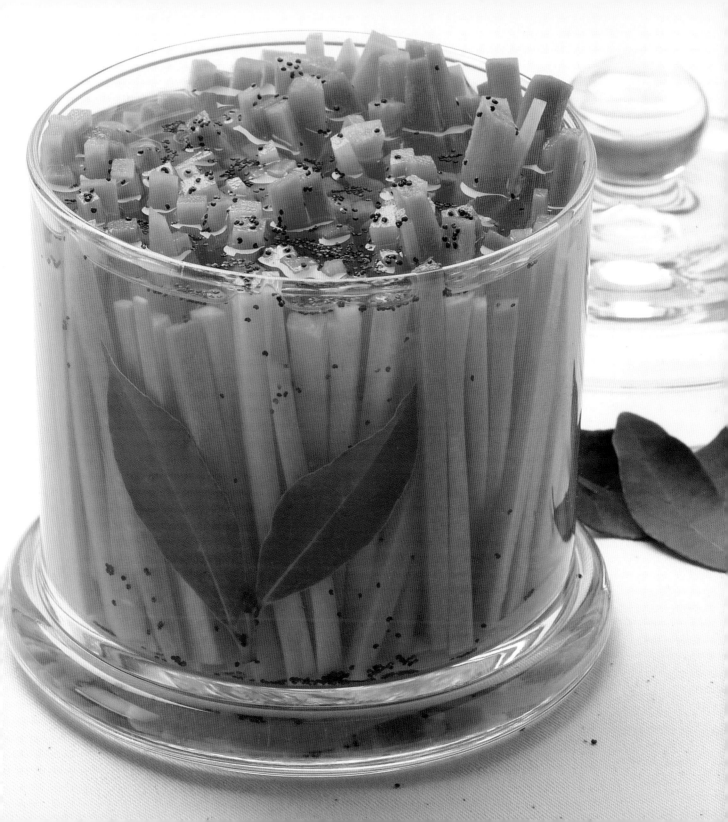

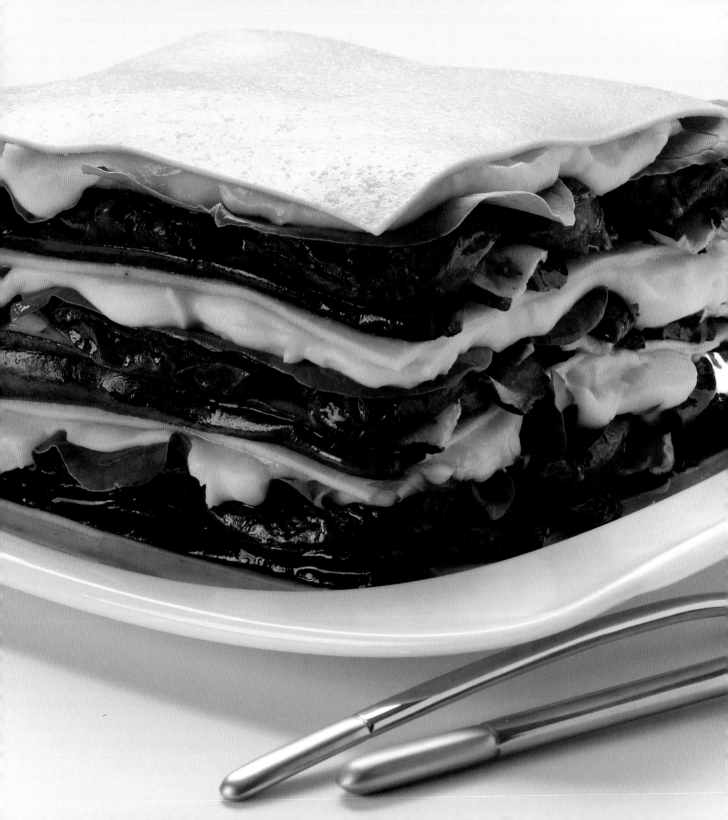

VEGETABLE LASAGNE STACK

Serves 2

This recipe is a quick no-bake alternative to vegetarian lasagne. The spinach is used raw however the hot vegetables and sauce will lightly wilt the leaves.

50g (2oz) unsalted butter
50g (2oz) plain flour
¼ cup (60ml/2fl oz) white wine
200ml (6fl oz) low-fat milk
50g (2oz) fresh parmesan cheese, grated

1 baby eggplant (aubergine), washed and cut into quarters
1 zucchini (courgette), washed, quartered
2 branches cherry truss tomatoes, washed

3 cloves garlic
200g (6½oz) fresh lasagne sheets
1 tablespoon olive oil
30 baby spinach leaves, washed and dried

Pre-heat oven to moderately slow, 160°C (325°F) Gas Mark 3. Melt the butter in a small saucepan, add the flour and mix into a paste. Add the wine and when it has been absorbed add the milk and cheese and stir until smooth. Coat all the vegetables except the spinach with olive oil and cook in the oven for 30 minutes. Cut the lasagne sheets into eight 10cm (4ins) squares then blanch for 3 minutes in boiling water. Remove from the water using a slotted spoon. Place in a bowl and coat with olive oil to prevent them from sticking.

Place 1 lasagne sheet on a plate, cover with a layer of hot vegetables, a layer of spinach and then the white sauce. Repeat process to create 4 layers on two separate plates.

Note: Packet or tinned parmesan cheese can be substituted but fresh will give much better flavour.

CORN AND CRAB OMELETTE TOPPED WITH WATERCRESS SALAD

Serves 2

4 eggs
100ml (6fl oz) milk
200g (6½oz) tinned corn kernels, drained
100g (3½oz) crab meat
1 bunch tarragon, leaves washed and
   picked, chopped

Sea salt and freshly ground black pepper
50g (2oz) unsalted butter
1 small bunch watercress, leaves washed
   and picked
1 tablespoon verjuice
1 tablespoon extra virgin olive oil

Whisk the eggs, milk, corn, crab meat, tarragon and a little salt and pepper in a bowl until combined.

Heat an omelette pan to a low heat, add the butter and when melted pour in the egg mixture and cook for 4 minutes. Finish cooking under the grill for a further 6 minutes. Put the watercress in a bowl and coat with verjuice and the extra virgin olive oil. Top the omelette with the dressed watercress and serve.

Note: For a healthier option use low-fat milk. Verjuice is a non-fermented green grape juice; you can substitute fresh lemon juice if you prefer.

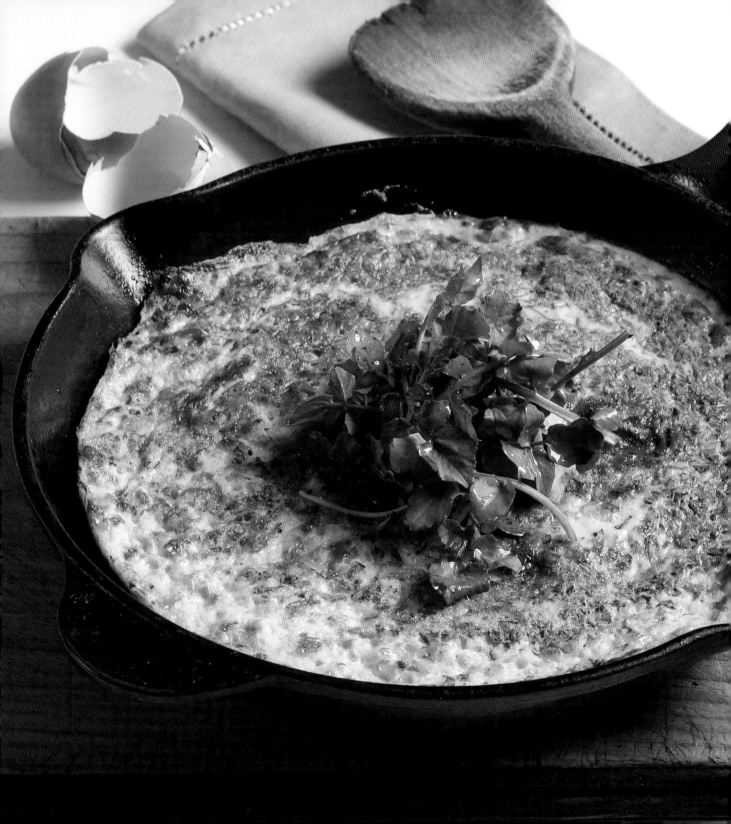

MOONG DAHL SALAD

This is a refreshing light salad and makes a wonderful accompaniment to hot curries.

70g (2½ oz) dried Moong Dahl (split mung beans)
2 tablespoons lemon juice
⅓ cup (80ml/2½fl oz) extra virgin olive oil
1 tablespoon yellow mustard seeds
1 tablespoon garam masala powder
1 bird's-eye chilli, sliced
Sea salt
2 medium carrots, peeled and grated
1 Spanish onion, sliced
½ bunch coriander (cilantro) leaves, washed and picked
½ bunch mint, washed and picked
¼ cup coconut, shredded

Put the mung beans in a bowl, cover with cold water and leave to soak overnight. The next day, drain and rinse under fresh running water.

Make the dressing by combining the lemon juice, oil, mustard seeds, garam masala, and chilli in a bowl. Add salt to taste. Place the beans, carrots, onion, coriander, mint and coconut in a serving bowl, drizzle with dressing and serve immediately.

Note: Mong dahl are split mung beans and are available from Asian grocers and the Asian sections of large supermarkets. You can replace the split mung beans with the common dried mung bean available from any supermarket. Garam masala is a spice blend of cardamom, Indian bay leaves, black pepper, cumin, coriander and cinnamon. It is available at most supermarkets. Bird's-eye chilli is very hot; if you prefer a milder taste remove the seeds before slicing the chilli.

CARROT AND GINGER SOUP

Serves 2

1 tablespoon olive oil
1kg (2lbs) carrots, peeled and diced
2 onions, roughly diced
2 cloves garlic, minced
2 tablespoons fresh ginger, minced

1 litre (1¾ pints) chicken stock
1 tablespoon honey
¼ cup (60ml/2fl oz) natural yoghurt
Sea salt and freshly ground black pepper

Heat the olive oil in a large saucepan and sauté the carrots, onions, garlic and ginger.
Add the chicken stock and honey and simmer for 20 minutes.
Put in a food processor and blend until a puree. Season to taste with salt and pepper.
Top with a dollop of yoghurt and serve with warm, crusty bread.

Note: Homemade chicken stock is best but reduced-salt packet chicken stock can be substituted.

QUICK WAYS WITH VEGETABLES

- Shred a red cabbage and cook in 2 cups (500ml/16fl oz) red wine vinegar, ¼ cup orange marmalade and 1 teaspoon caraway seeds for about 10 minutes or until caramelised.

- Roast pumpkin wedges in olive oil and serve drizzled with a little maple syrup and a sprinkle of sesame seeds.

- Chopped fresh thyme and sliced garlic gives green beans a sensational flavour. Powdered thyme can be substituted for fresh.

- A dollop of pesto gives halved and steamed yellow squash a touch of class.

- Broccoli leaves and turnip leaves are a taste sensation. Lightly steam for 4 minutes. Serve with a splash of extra virgin olive oil. These winter greens are available at greengrocers.

QUICK WAYS WITH FROZEN PEAS

- In soup: Sauté 1 onion, 2 sliced garlic cloves and 500g (1lb) frozen peas. Add 1 litre (1¾ pints) homemade or reduced-salt packet chicken stock. Simmer for 30 minutes. Puree and serve with a sprinkle of chopped mint.

- Mushy: Sauté 1 onion, 2 sliced garlic cloves and 500g (1lb) frozen peas. Add 200ml (6fl oz) homemade or reduced-salt packet chicken stock. Puree together. Delicious served on toast.

- In a salad: Blanch peas in boiling water for just a few seconds. Refresh with cool water. Use sprinkled in garden salads.

QUICK WAYS WITH ASPARAGUS

Trim woody ends off asparagus and:

- Cook on the barbecue (grill) for 3 minutes. Dress with olive oil and a sprinkle of sea salt.

- Roll in flour, dip in beaten egg and roll in grated parmesan cheese.

- Cook in moderate oven for 15 minutes or until golden. Can be served as a side dish or as a snack.

- Lightly blanch in boiling water for 4 minutes. Serve with a splash of extra virgin olive oil and lemon juice.

QUICK WAYS WITH CAPSICUMS (BELL PEPPERS)

- Coat red capsicums in light olive oil and barbecue (grill) whole until slightly blackened. Place in a bowl of cool water, peel, cut in half and remove seeds. Drizzle with a little extra virgin olive oil. These go well with meat, fish, chicken and salads.

- Slice red or green capsicums, toss with flaked almonds, coriander and chopped mint leaves. Sprinkle with lemon zest and dress with a dash of extra virgin olive oil. Serve with barbecued meat or a spicy lamb dish.

- Cut capsicums in half, remove seeds and fill with chicken mince and finely sliced garlic mixed with a little cooked brown rice. Top with a teaspoon of chilli jam. Put in an ovenproof dish half-filled with bottled tomato puree. Spoon some puree over the capsicums a couple of times when cooking. Cook for 30 minutes in a moderate oven.

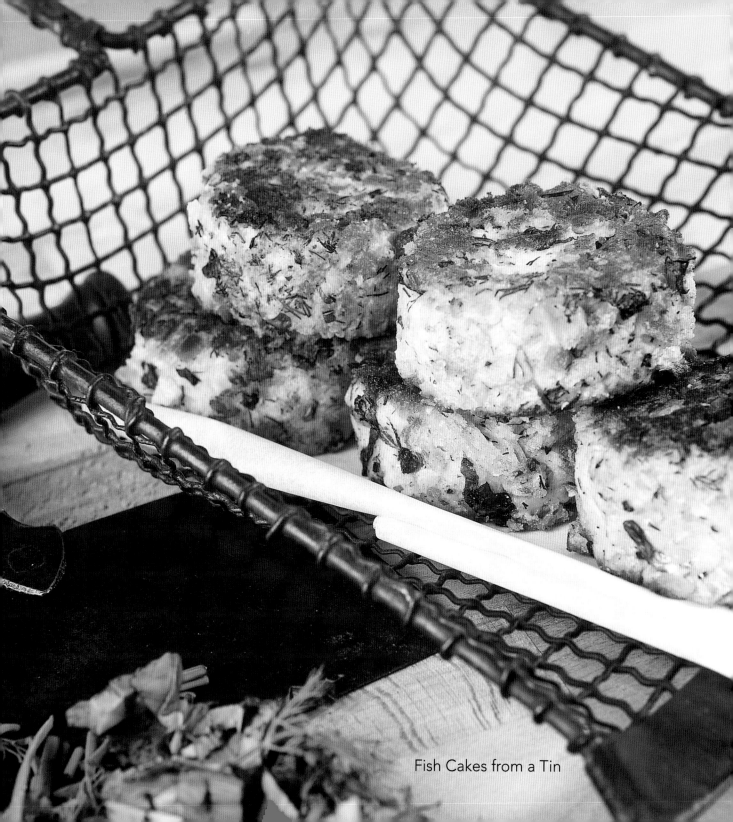

Fish Cakes from a Tin

Six

MEALS IN A HURRY

It's amazing how many times I find myself feeding hoards of friends in a strange kitchen and having to make do with whatever produce is on hand—just because I'm a chef people often turn to me for a quick creation.

Meals made in a hurry never have to look like it though. If you have a tin of salmon or tuna in your pantry or some eggs in the refrigerator you can create something delicious without too much trouble. For instance, frittata can be made in no time at all using eggs and leftover vegetables. My speciality, Spinach and Olive Frittata, is quick and easy to make and everyone loves it.

I use a French cast iron pan for cooking frittata because cast iron distributes heat so evenly.

FISH CAKES FROM A TIN

Serves 2

Serve with watercress lightly coated in finest quality extra virgin olive oil and for pure indulgence a dollop of hollandaise sauce.

150g (2oz) potatoes, diced
200g (6½oz) tinned salmon, drained
Sea salt and freshly ground black pepper
1 bunch parsley, washed and chopped
2 tablespoons fresh parmesan cheese,
grated
1 cup breadcrumbs
1 cup flour
2 eggs, lightly beaten
2 tablespoons light olive oil

Peel the potatoes and from a cold water start, boil until they are tender, drain and mash. Mix the salmon, potato, a little salt and pepper and half the parsley until combined. Mould the fish mix into round cakes.
Mix the breadcrumbs, parmesan and the remainder of the parsley together. Roll the fish cakes in the flour and dip them in the beaten egg before rolling in the breadcrumb mix. Heat the oil in the frying pan and bring to a medium heat and gently fry the fish cakes for 4 minutes on each side or until golden brown. Remove from the pan and rest on absorbent paper before serving (see picture page 144).

Note: For a healthier option omit the hollandaise sauce. Don't add butter or milk when mashing the potatoes as it's best to keep the fish mixture fairly dry to prevent the fish cakes from breaking up when frying.

SALMON WITH DILL MAYONNAISE ON SOURDOUGH

This dish makes a perfect light lunch or a delicious snack. Fresh poached salmon can be substituted if you prefer.

200g (6½oz) tinned salmon, drained
½ bunch dill, leaves washed, picked and
    chopped
2 tablespoons homemade mayonnaise
    (See recipe Chapter 4, From the Ocean)

1 teaspoon salted baby capers
4 thick slices sourdough bread
1 tablespoon extra virgin olive oil

Mix the salmon, dill, mayonnaise and capers until combined. Toast the sourdough, drizzle with the oil, top with the salmon mixture and serve.

Note: Store-bought mayonnaise can be substituted but it will not have as good a flavour as homemade mayonnaise. For a healthier option use low-fat mayonnaise.

SALMON AND CHICKPEA SALAD

Serves 2

200g (6½oz) tinned chickpeas
100g (3½oz) tinned salmon, drained
1 Spanish onion, peeled and sliced
1 punnet cherry tomatoes, washed and
  cut in halves

1 bunch flat leaf parsley, leaves washed
  and picked
Juice and grated zest of 1 lemon
1 tablespoon extra virgin olive oil
Sea salt and freshly ground black pepper

Drain and wash the chickpeas in cold water and toss with all the other ingredients in
a bowl. Season to taste with salt and pepper and serve.

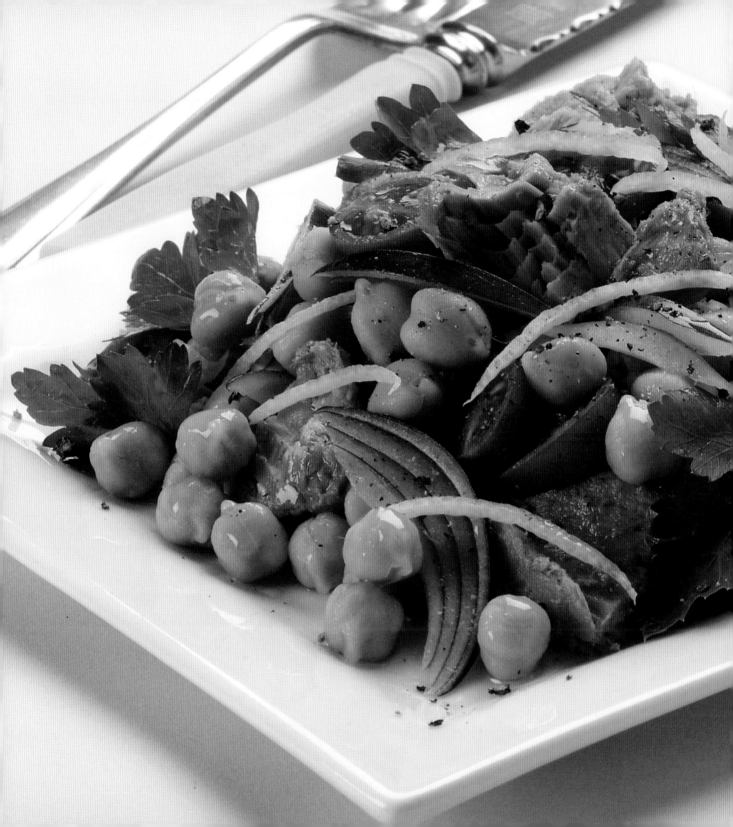

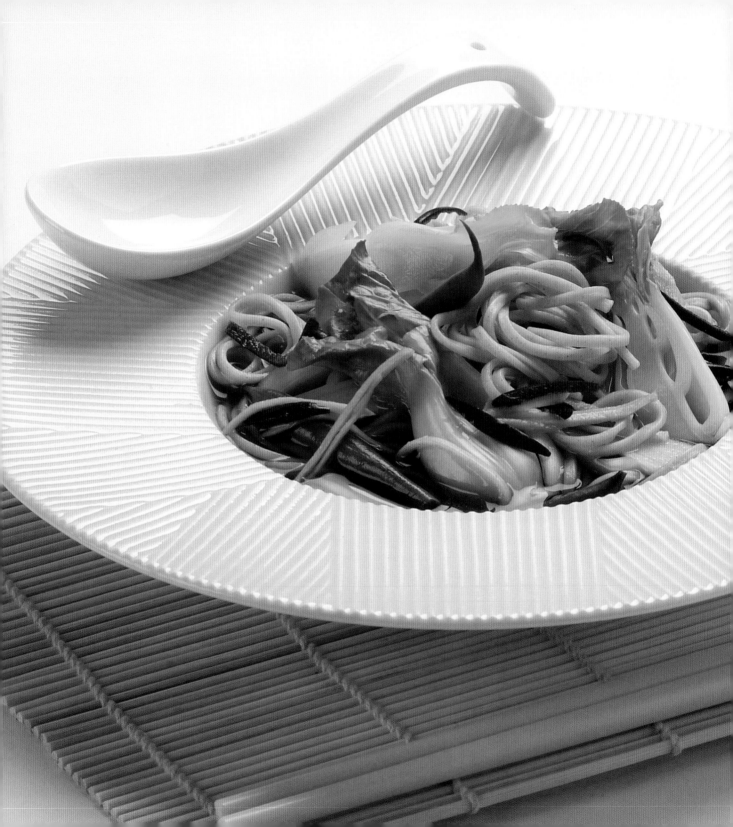

SOBA NOODLES
WITH WARM JAPANESE DRESSING

Serves 2

200g (6½oz) soba noodles
1 chilli, finely sliced
1 teaspoon fresh ginger, minced
1 cup (250ml/8fl oz) water
1 tablespoon miso paste

1 tablespoon maple syrup
1 tablespoon soy sauce
2 baby bok choy (pak choi), cut in halves
100g (3½oz) green beans

Boil the soba noodles for 15 minutes or until tender, drain and put equal portions in 2 bowls.

Sauté the chilli and ginger for 2 minutes then add the water, miso paste, maple syrup and soy sauce and stir until dissolved.

Blanch the bok choy and green beans in boiling water for 4 minutes, drain and spoon over the noodles. Pour over the hot dressing and serve.

Note: Soba noodles are Japanese noodles and bok choy are small, green Chinese vegetables. Both are available at Asian grocers and most supermarkets. I always keep a packet in my pantry but spaghetti can be substituted.

COUSCOUS WITH PUMPKIN, SPINACH AND FETA

Serves 2 or 4 as a side dish

½ butternut pumpkin, peeled and diced large
2 tablespoons light olive oil
Sea salt
1½ cups couscous
2 tablespoons raisins

½ bunch basil, leaves washed and chopped
50g (2oz) baby spinach, washed and dried
100g (3½oz) reduced-fat feta, diced

Pre-heat oven to moderate, 180°C (350°F) Gas Mark 4. Coat the pumpkin in olive oil and sprinkle with a little salt.

Place on a baking tray and cook for 15–20 minutes or until tender.

Put the couscous and raisins in a heatproof bowl and just cover with boiling water. Use cling wrap to cover the bowl for three minutes or until the water has been fully absorbed, then fluff the couscous with a fork and mix through the pumpkin, basil, spinach and feta.

Note: 100g (3½oz) of frozen spinach can be substituted for the baby spinach in this recipe.

LINGUINE WITH CAPERS, SMOKED SALMON AND ROCKET

Serves 2

200g (6½oz) linguine
2 tablespoons light olive oil
1 Spanish onion, sliced
1 clove garlic, sliced
100g (3½oz) smoked salmon

1 tablespoon salted capers
1 bunch rocket, washed and stalks
 removed
1 tablespoon extra virgin olive oil

Boil the linguine in salted water for 15 minutes or until al dente, drain but do not refresh in cold water as this will slow down the cooking process.

Heat the light olive oil in a large frying pan, sauté the onion and garlic, then add the linguine, smoked salmon, capers and rocket.

Stir until all ingredients are mixed together. Serve with a drizzle of extra virgin olive oil.

SPINACH AND OLIVE FRITTATA

Serves 2

This can be served hot or cold.

Olive oil spray
1 potato, diced
5 eggs
200ml (6fl oz) milk
Sea salt and freshly ground black pepper

50g (2oz) fresh parmesan cheese, grated
50g (2oz) baby spinach, washed and dried
2 tablespoons kalamata olives, pitted
6 cherry tomatoes, washed

Pre-heat oven to moderate, 180°C (350°F) Gas Mark 4. Spray a 20cm (8ins) cast iron pan or ceramic dish with olive oil and put to one side.
Boil the diced potatoes until tender. Whisk the eggs and milk together in a bowl and season to taste with salt and pepper. Gently stir in the cheese, potatoes, spinach, olives and tomatoes. Spoon into the pan and cook for 20 minutes.

Note: For a healthier option use low-fat milk. For a special occasion substitute cream for a richer frittata.

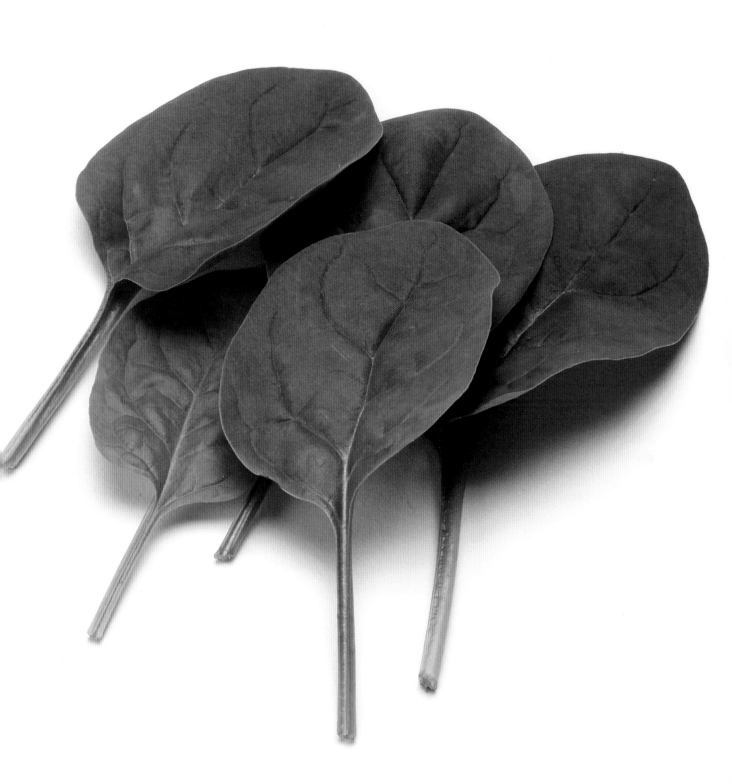

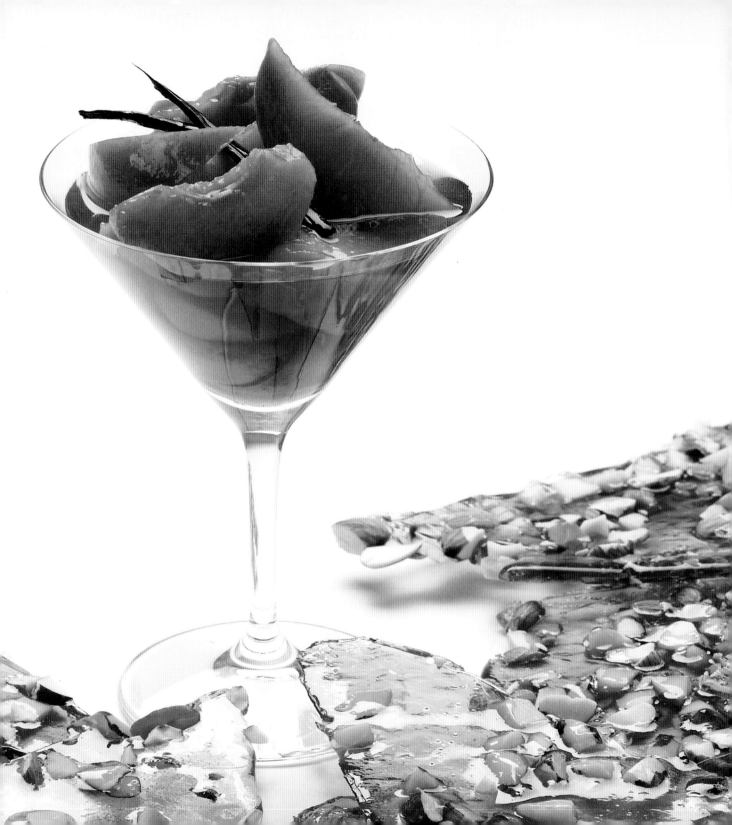

Seven

SOMETHING SWEET

No fine meal is complete without dessert. It can be the most sinful of chocolate concoctions or the freshest strawberries with a splash of balsamic vinegar.

Fresh fruit always makes the perfect dessert and in the interests of your eye health you should eat it daily. However, that doesn't mean you can't indulge now and then because there are times when an occasion calls for a dessert that's a little bit special.

What I enjoy most about making desserts is the sounds they create. Put a dessert in front of someone and there they are—aaah...hmmmm....oooooh—the sounds of ecstasy, anticipation, approval and indulgence. I find it soothing to make sweet things that bring so much pleasure to people of all ages.

As a romantic I love working with chocolate; the fact that it has had a long association with love appeals to me. Centuries ago, French doctors prescribed it for patients with emotional disorders, including women suffering from a broken heart.

I have put together some relatively healthy dessert options, including something chocolatey of course, that will still keep the sweetest tooth satisfied. My chocolate sorbet is an absolute sensual overload—extraordinarily rich but quite unbelievably low in fat.

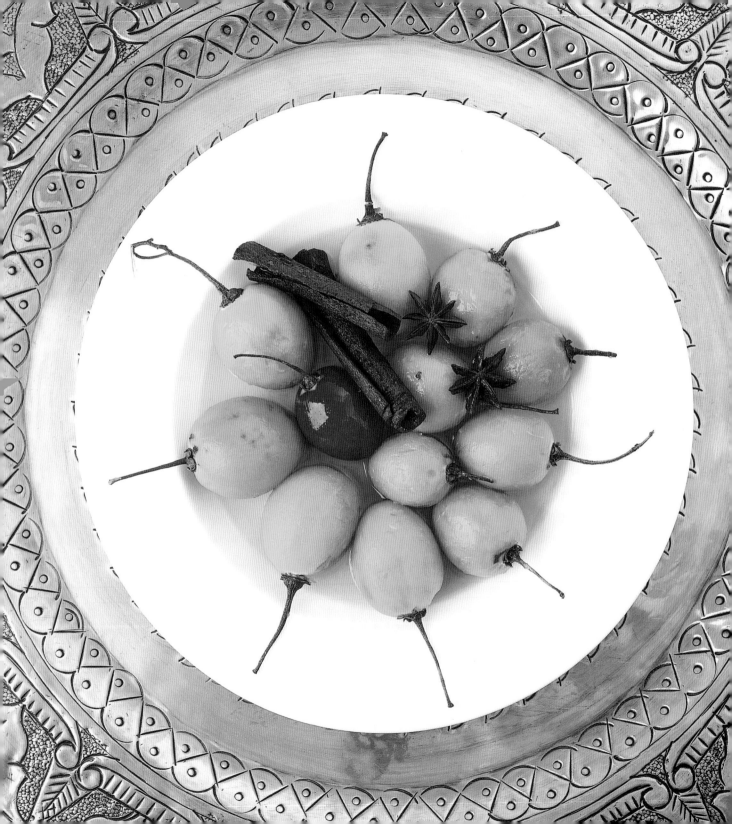

WINTER TAMARILLOS WITH ROSE WATER

Serves 4

8 tamarillos
2 cups (500ml/16fl oz) water
2 star anise
1 cinnamon quill

¼ cup (60ml/2fl oz) rose water
200g (6½ oz) white sugar
250ml (8oz) double cream (optional)

Using a sharp knife gently score a cross on the bottom of each tamarillo.
Simmer the water, spices, rose water and sugar in a saucepan for 10 minutes to create a sugar syrup.
Plunge the tamarillos into the syrup and poach for 7 minutes. Remove and peel.
Serve with the warm syrup and cream.

BLOOD ORANGE JELLY
WITH CITRUS AND MINT SALAD

Serves 4

5 gelatine leaves
7 blood oranges, juiced (makes
   700ml/1¼ pints, see note)
½ cup caster sugar
1 cinnamon quill

Citrus and Mint Salad
1 ruby red grapefruit, skin and seeds
   removed, cut and diced
1 navel orange, skin and seeds removed,
   cut and diced
½ bunch mint, leaves washed, picked
   and finely chopped

Soak the gelatine in cold water for 5 minutes or until soft. Remove, squeeze out any excess water from the gelatine and put on a plate.

Simmer the orange juice, sugar and cinnamon for 5 minutes. Add the gelatine and stir until dissolved. Remove from the heat and strain through a fine sieve. Pour the mixture into 4 small moulds. (If you don't have any moulds small coffee cups make good substitutes.) Allow to set in the refrigerator for a minimum of 3 hours.

To make the citrus salad, mix the diced orange, mint and grapefruit in a small bowl. Unmould the jelly by quickly placing the mould in boiling water and then inverting on to individual plates. Serve with the citrus salad.

Note: When setting desserts, gelatine leaves give a fail-proof result. They are available at all good delicatessens and come in 2g and 5g sheets. If blood oranges are out of season, tinned blood orange juice can be substituted.

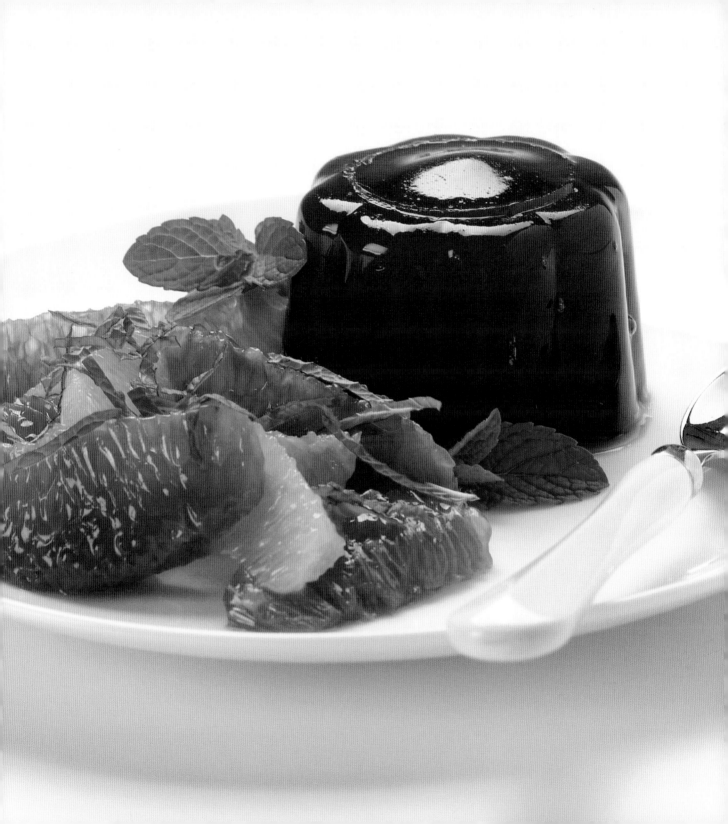

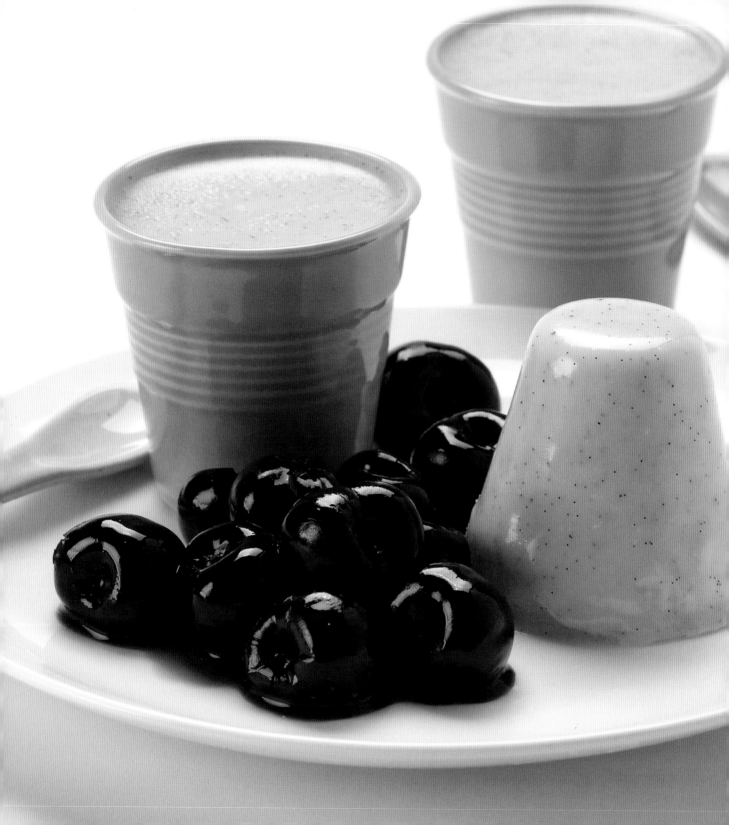

YOGHURT PANNA COTTA WITH POACHED CHERRIES

Serves 4

3 gelatine leaves
375ml (12fl oz) cream
2 tablespoons natural
  yoghurt
1 vanilla bean, split and
  scraped

1 cinnamon stick
1 star anise
½ cup caster sugar

Poached Cherries
1 cup caster sugar
1 cup (250ml/8fl oz) water
500g (1lb) cherries,
  washed and pitted

Soak the gelatine in cold water for 5 minutes or until soft. Remove and squeeze out excess water from the gelatine and put on a plate.

Bring the cream, yoghurt, vanilla, cinnamon, star anise and sugar to the simmer for 4 minutes. Stir in the gelatine until dissolved. Remove from the heat and strain through a fine sieve.

Pour the mixture into 4 small moulds. (If you don't have any moulds small coffee cups make good substitutes.) Allow to set in the refrigerator for a minimum of 3 hours but for best results leave overnight.

When ready to serve, quickly dip the moulds in boiling water and turn out the panna cottas on a plate.

To poach the cherries, simmer sugar and water in a saucepan for 5 minutes, add the cherries and continue to simmer for a further 5 minutes. Allow to cool and serve with the panna cottas.

Note: For a healthier option use reduced-fat cream

MANGO AND STRAWBERRIES TOPPED WITH LIME AND MANGO GRANITA

Serves 4

300ml (10fl oz) mango nectar
Juice of 2 limes
220g (7oz) caster sugar
60ml (2fl oz) honey-infused vodka

2 mango cheeks, skin removed
1 punnet strawberries, washed, tops
   removed and cut in half
Additional honey-infused vodka

To prepare the granita, simmer the mango nectar, lime juice, sugar and vodka in a small saucepan for 5 minutes. Pour into a shallow metal tray (20 x 25 x 5cm/8 x 10 x 2ins) and cool before putting in the freezer for 30 minutes or until ice crystals start to form. Rake the crystals with a fork to prevent them forming a solid mass. Repeat this process twice. When you serve the granita it should look like fluffy crystals.
Use a large tablespoon to scoop out the flesh from the mango cheeks then slice and arrange them in martini glasses or dessert dishes. Add the strawberries, top with the granita and finish with a splash of the additional honey-infused vodka.

Note: Honey-infused vodka is available from most bottle shops. If you have trouble finding it, make your own by adding ¼ cup of honey to 500ml (16fl oz) of vodka.

ROSÉ AND RASPBERRY JELLY

Serves 2

This dessert looks terrific served in martini glasses with a dollop of mascarpone on top and fresh biscotti on the side.

4 gelatine leaves
750ml (24fl oz) rosé wine
Grated zest of 1 orange
1 punnet raspberries, washed

Soak the gelatine in cold water for 5 minutes or until soft. Remove, squeeze out any excess water from the gelantine and put on a plate.
Place the wine and orange zest in a saucepan and boil for 5 minutes or until only about two-thirds of the liquid is remaining. Add the gelatine and stir until dissolved. Remove from heat and strain through a fine sieve. Spoon the raspberries and enough liquid to cover them into two elegant glasses and allow to set in the refrigerator for one hour.
Leave the remainder of the liquid jelly standing at room temperature. Remove the glasses of set jelly from the refrigerator and top with the liquid. Return to the refrigerator for a further 3 hours or until set.

Note: Jelly is set in two layers to prevent raspberries from floating to the top.

PEARS IN RED WINE

Serve with a scoop of vanilla ice cream or for special occasions add a dollop of mascarpone.

1 bottle claret (750ml/24fl oz)
2 cups (500ml/16fl oz) water
1 cup white sugar

1 vanilla pod, scraped
1 cinnamon quill
6 beurre bosc pears, peeled and cored

Place the wine, water, sugar, vanilla and cinnamon quill in a large saucepan and simmer for 5 minutes or until the sugar has dissolved.
Place the pears in the liquid standing upright, the liquid should cover the pears. Simmer the pears for 10 minutes or until tender. Insert a skewer to test if they are cooked.
Remove from heat and chill in the poaching liquid in the refrigerator for one hour before serving.

Note: For a healthier option use reduced-fat vanilla ice cream.

APPLE AND RASPBERRY CRUMBLE

Serves 6

6 ripe, green apples, peeled and diced
125ml (4fl oz) water
1/3 cup caster sugar
1 punnet raspberries
100g (3½ oz) butter

1/3 cup honey
2 cups rolled oats
¼ cup sunflower seeds
¼ cup pumpkin seeds

Pre-heat oven to moderate, 180°C (350°F) Gas Mark 4.
Place the apples, water and sugar in a medium saucepan and simmer for 15 minutes.
Remove from the heat, fold in the raspberries and spoon into 6 ceramic bowls.
To make the crumble, melt the butter and honey in a small saucepan. Remove from heat, add the oats and seeds and mix together.
Completely cover the fruit with the mixture. Bake for 15 minutes or until golden brown.

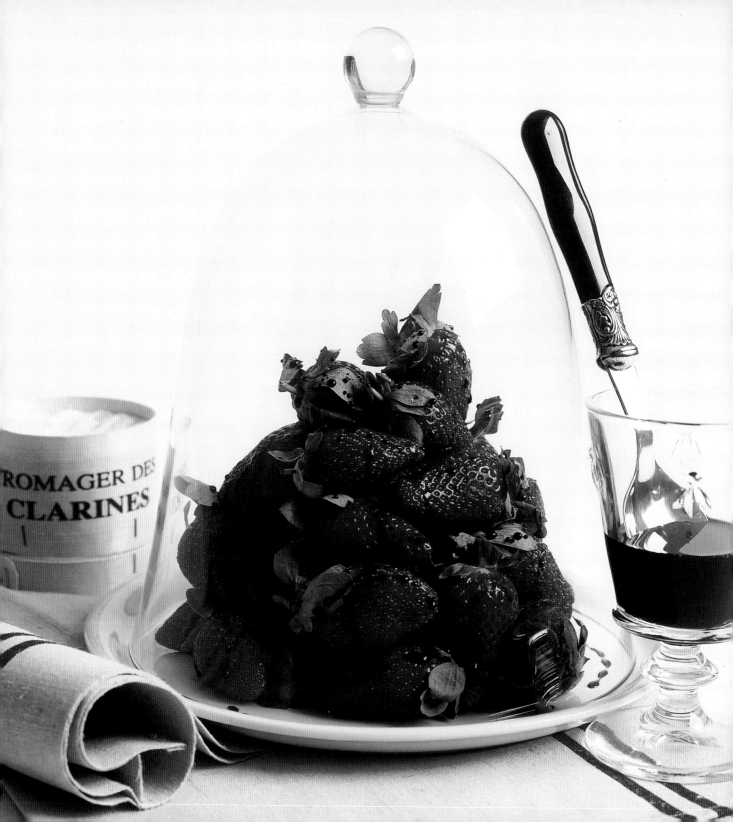

WHOLE STRAWBERRIES WITH BALSAMIC SYRUP

Serves 4

½ cup (125ml/4fl oz) balsamic vinegar
½ cup sugar
400g (13oz) strawberries

Place the vinegar and sugar in a small saucepan and stir.
Simmer, stirring continuously for 5 minutes or until a syrupy consistency is reached.
Arrange the strawberries on a cake stand or platter and drizzle with the balsamic syrup.

SUMMER STONE FRUIT SERVED WITH PRALINE

Serves 4

This goes beautifully with vanilla ice cream.

3 cups (750ml/24fl oz) water
1 cup caster sugar
1 vanilla bean, split and scraped
1 yellow nectarine
1 yellow peach
1 white peach
1 quantity of praline (See Chapter One, Snack Time for recipe)

Simmer the water, sugar and vanilla in a large saucepan for 5 minutes.
Using a small sharp knife lightly cut a cross at the bottom of each piece of fruit
and plunge into simmering liquid for 5 minutes or until the skin starts to peel away.
Remove the fruit with a slotted spoon and refresh in a bowl of cold water. Continue
to boil the sugar and water mixture for 7 minutes or until the liquid has reached a
syrupy consistency.
Peel the fruit and slice into quarters and divide evenly into four martini glasses.
Crumble the praline over the fruit and cover with the poaching liquid.

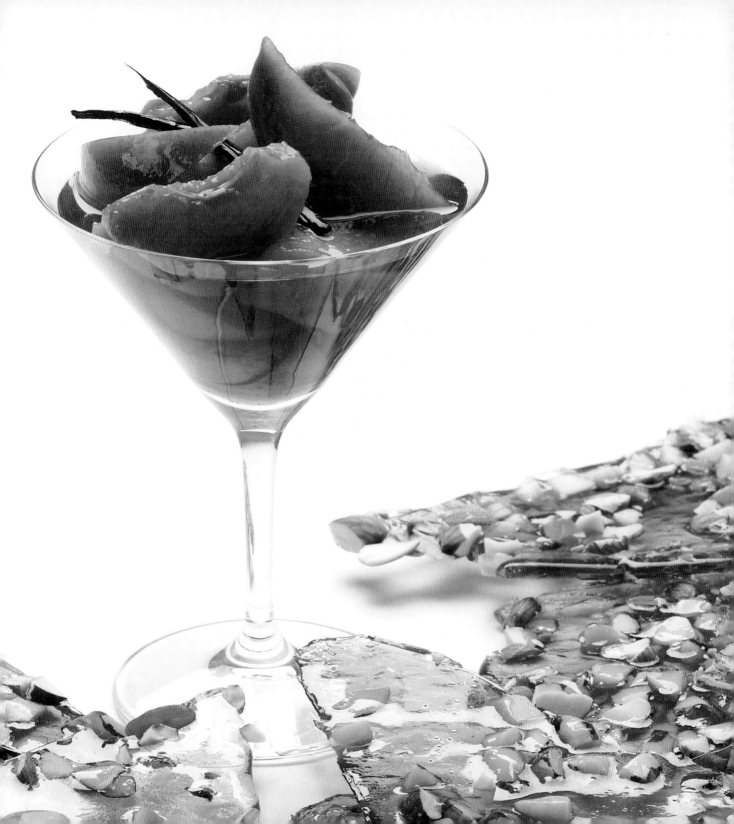

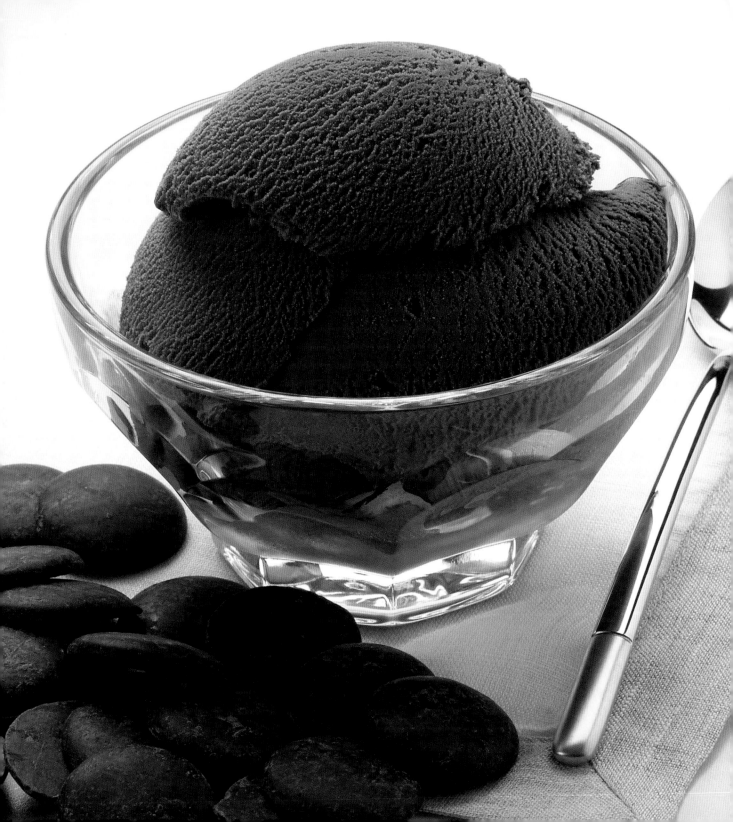

CHOCOLATE SORBET

Serves 4

240ml (8fl oz) full cream milk
200g (6½oz) Belgian chocolate buttons
150g (2oz) Dutch cocoa

900ml (30fl oz) full cream milk (additional)
500g (1lb) caster sugar

Bring the first smaller amount of milk to the boil. Remove from heat, add the chocolate buttons and stir until smooth and glossy.

Sift the cocoa into the second, larger amount of milk, add the sugar and whisk well until the cocoa is incorporated. Stir in the warm chocolate mix. Strain through a sieve removing any lumps to ensure a smooth, silky mixture.

Freeze in an ice cream maker as per manufacturer's instructions or alternatively pour the chocolate mixture into a flat rectangular freezer-proof container and place in the freezer for one hour. The sorbet mixture should be almost frozen when you take it out.

Spoon into a chilled food processor and quickly puree.

Pour into the freezer-proof container and cover with a fitted lid or cling wrap. Place in the freezer for at least six hours or overnight.

Eight

WHEN YOU'RE THIRSTY

An enjoyable drink can be alcoholic or non-alcoholic. Strawberry Lemonade and Sangria are both perfect to serve on a hot summer's day. Sangria is a marvellous thirst-quenching drink that goes particularly well with spicy food.

STRAWBERRY LEMONADE

Serves 4

6 lemons
300g (9½oz) caster sugar
350g (11oz) strawberries
Ice cubes, soda water or (if you prefer) champagne, to serve
100g (3½oz) strawberries to serve, optional

Using a zester, remove the rind from the lemons and put in a large bowl with the sugar and strawberries. Juice the lemons and stir the juice into the strawberry mixture. Add 1½ litres (2½ pints) of boiling water and mix well. Cool to room temperature and refrigerate overnight.
Strain the mixture through a coarse sieve and pour into sterilised bottles.
Serve over ice cubes and fresh strawberries in champagne glasses and top with soda or champagne.

Note: Strawberry Lemonade will keep refrigerated for up to a week.

SANGRIA

I like to serve sangria in red wine glasses.

1 cup (250ml/8fl oz) orange juice
½ cup (125ml/4fl oz) lemon juice
½ cup sugar
1 bottle light-bodied red wine (750ml /24fl oz), well chilled
½ orange sliced
½ ripe green apple, sliced

In a medium-sized saucepan bring the orange juice, lemon juice and sugar to the simmer for 3 minutes. Stir until the sugar is dissolved then allow to cool.
Pour the red wine into a large jug or bowl, add the cooled juices, sliced fruit and some ice cubes.

Nine

NUTRITION AND EYE HEALTH

While there is no cure for macular degeneration, there are measures that can be taken to optimise eye health which may slow down the progression of the disease. Diet plays an important role in good eye health. Studies have shown that macular degeneration responds to antioxidants, vitamins, minerals and other nutrients. However, any changes in diet and lifestyle should be undertaken in consultation with a doctor. Be aware that some foods may interact with prescription drugs and may not suit some medical conditions.

ANTIOXIDANTS FOR EYE HEALTH

Antioxidants are important to our health and are found in the foods we eat. When cells turn food and oxygen into energy they also produce 'free radicals'. These are thought to be a contributing factor in the cause of macular degeneration and other diseases. Free radicals can be neutralised by antioxidants.

ANTIOXIDANTS FOR EYE HEALTH

		Daily Intake*
Lutein and Zeaxanthin	Lutein is a particularly important antioxidant for eye health. It is present in high concentrations in the macula and needs to be frequently replenished. It is found in particularly high levels in dark green leafy vegetables such as spinach.	6mg**
Vitamin C	Vitamin C is necessary for normal structure and function of connective tissue. Found in citrus fruits, papaya and rockmelon.	45mg*
Vitamin E	Vitamin E is necessary for cell protection from the damage caused by free radicals. Found in nuts, wheat germ, whole grains and green leafy vegetables.	7-10mg*
Zinc	Zinc contributes to the normal structure of skin and normal wound healing and contributes to a healthy immune system. Found in meat, seafood (especially oysters), seeds, nuts and whole grains.	8-14mg*

OTHER NUTRIENTS

		Daily Intake
Selenium	Selenium is necessary for cell protection from some types of damage caused by free radicals.	60-70µg*
Omega-3	Omega-3 supports the normal development of the brain, eyes and nerves.	0.9-1.6g

Where a range is shown this indicates differing intakes required by men and women.
* Intake values prescribed by the National Health and Medical Research Council (NHMRC).
** There is no standard intake for lutein; 6mg is considered an acceptable daily intake.

Daily intake refers to the amount of specific nutrients considered adequate to meet the nutritional requirements of healthy people. It is formulated as a way to help prevent nutritional deficiency diseases in healthy people and it should be remembered that it does not address the special needs of people who smoke, are in ill health or are on medication, for example.

Below is the nutrient content information for some common foods.

Vegetables	Lutein & Zeaxanthin (mg/100g 3½oz)	Vitamin C (mg/100g 3½oz)	Vitamin E (mg/100g 3½oz)	Zinc (mg/100g 3½oz)
Kale	18.2	41	0.85	0.24
Spinach	11.3	9.8	2.1	0.76
Peas	2.4	40	0.13	1.20
Lettuce, Cos	2.3	24	0.13	0.23
Broccoli	1.1	65	1.5	0.45
Pumpkin	1.0	4.7	0.8	0.23
Corn	0.9	6.8	0.07	0.45
Brussels Sprouts	0.9	62	0.43	0.33
Beans, green	0.7	9.7	0.45	0.25
Asparagus	0.8	7.7	1.5	0.60
Capsicum (sweet pepper/bell pepper)	0.5	127	1.6	0.25
Celery	0.4	6.1	0.35	0.14
Carrots	0.3	3.6	1.0	0.20
Lettuce, Iceberg	0.3	2.8	0.18	0.15
Tomato (raw)	0.1	12.7	0.54	0.17

Fruit	Lutein & Zeaxanthin (mg/100g 3½oz)	Vitamin C (mg/100g 3½oz)	Vitamin E (mg/100g 3½oz)	Zinc (mg/100g 3½oz)
Tangerine	0.14	27	0.20	0.07
Orange	0.13	53	0.18	0.07
Papaya	0.08	62	0.73	0.07
Peach	0.09	6.6	0.73	0.17
Rockmelon (cantaloupe)	0.03	37	0.05	0.18
Apple	0.03	4.6	0.18	0.04
Watermelon	0.01	8.1	0.05	0.10
Grapefruit	0.01	37	0	0.07

Other	Lutein & Zeaxanthin mg	Vitamin C mg	Vitamin E mg	Zinc mg
Egg (per 60g (2oz) egg)	0.27	0	0.97	1.1

Source: US Department of Agriculture (USDA) www.nal.usda.gov

Nuts	Selenium µg/100g (3½oz)	Vitamin E mg/100g (3½oz)	Zinc mg/100g (3½oz)
Almonds	2.8	25.9	3.6
Brazil	1917	5.7	4.1
Cashew	20	0.9	5.5
Pecan	3.8	1.4	3.9
Pine Nut	0.7	9.3	5.3
Pistachio	7.0	2.3	2.3

Source: www.nutsforlife.com.au

Fresh Fish	Total Fat g/100g (3½oz)	Sat. Fat g/100g (3½oz)	Poly. Fat g/100g (3½oz)	Omega-3 g/100g (3½oz)	Mono. Fat g/100g (3½oz)	Zinc mg/100g (3½oz)
Salmon, Atlantic	15.7	4.4	2.9	1.8	6.3	0.4
Trout, Rainbow	8.4	2.5	2	1.5	2.7	0.8
Bream	5.4	1.7	1.3	1.0	1.8	0.8
Tuna	1.0	0.2	0.3	0.2	1.2	0.5
Flathead	1.2	0.3	0.3	0.2	0.2	0.7

Source: www.foodstandards.gov.au

Other Fresh Seafood	Total Fat g/100g (3½oz)	Sat. Fat g/100g (3½oz)	Poly. Fat g/100g (3½oz)	Omega-3 g/100g (3½oz)	Mono. Fat g/100g (3½oz)	Zinc mg/100g (3½oz)
Oysters	2.4	0.8	0.7	0.5	0.2	47.9
Prawns (shrimp)	0.9	0.2	0.2	0.2	0.1	1.6

Source: www.foodstandards.gov.au

Ten

THE FACTS ABOUT MACULAR DEGENERATION

What is macular degeneration?

The macula is the central part of the retina, the light sensitive tissue at the back of the eye. The retina processes all visual images. It is responsible for your ability to read, recognise faces, drive and see colours clearly. You are reading this text using your macula. Macular degeneration causes progressive macular damage resulting in loss of central vision but the peripheral vision is not affected.

How common is macular degeneration?

Macular degeneration is the leading cause of blindness* and severe vision loss in Australia. One in seven people over the age of 50 years is affected in some way and the incidence increases with age.

What are the types of macular degeneration?

There are two types of macular degeneration. The 'dry' form results in a gradual loss of central vision. The 'wet' form is characterised by a sudden loss of vision and is caused by abnormal blood vessels growing into the retina. Immediate medical treatment is essential if symptoms occur.

* Legal blindness

What are the risk factors for macular degeneration?

There are three major risk factors for developing Macular Degeneration:

- Age: it affects 1 in 7 Australians over the age of 50 and the incidence increases with age.[1]
- Family History: it is hereditary, with a 50% chance of developing it if a direct family history of the disease is present.[2]
- Smoking: studies have shown that those who smoke are 3 times more likely to develop macular degeneration, and smokers may also develop the disease 10 years earlier than non-smokers.[3-4]

What treatments are available for macular degeneration?

Treatment options are dependent on the stage and type of the disease. Current treatments aim to keep the best vision for as long as possible and in some cases may potentially provide visual improvement, but there is presently no cure. Early detection is vital in saving sight.

Key symptoms may include one or more of the following:

- Difficulty with reading or any other activity that requires fine vision.
- Distortion, where straight lines appear wavy or bent.
- Distinguishing faces becomes a problem.
- Dark patches or empty spaces appear in the centre of your vision.

The need for increased illumination, sensitivity to glare, decreased night vision and poor colour sensitivity may also indicate that there is something wrong. If you experience any of these symptoms contact your eye care specialist immediately.

Early detection is important!

The early detection of any form of macular degeneration is crucial because the earlier you seek treatment, the more likely you are to have a better outcome compared to those who wait. Macular degeneration can cause many different symptoms. Difficulty with your vision should not be dismissed as part of just 'getting older'. In its early stages, macular degeneration may not be noticed but it can be detected in an eye test before any visual symptoms occur. Early detection can allow you to take steps to slow the progression of the disease.

Eye health checklist:

- Have your eyes tested and make sure the macula is checked.
- Don't smoke.
- Keep a healthy lifestyle, control your weight and exercise regularly.
- Eat a healthy, well-balanced diet. Limit your intake of fats, eat fish two or three times a week, eat dark green leafy vegetables and fresh fruit daily and a handful of nuts a week.
- In consultation with your doctor, consider a suitable supplement.
- Provide adequate protection for your eyes from sunlight exposure, especially when young.

[1] Van Newkirk MR et al. Ophthalmology 2000; 107: 1593–1600

[2] Smith W, Mitchell P. Aust NZ J Ohthalmol 1998; 26: 203–6

[3] Thornton J et al. Eye 2005; 19: 935–44

[4] Mitchell P et al. Arch Ophthalmol 2002; 120: 1357–63

WEIGHTS AND MEASURES CONVERSION CHART

Dry Measures

15g	½oz
30g	1oz
60g	2oz
90g	3oz
125g	4oz (¼ lb)
155g	5oz
180g	6oz
220g	7oz
250g	8oz (½ lb)
280g	9oz
315g	10oz
345g	11oz
375g	12oz
410g	13oz
440g	14oz
470g	15oz
500g	16oz (1lb)
750g	24oz (1½ lb)
1kg	32oz (2lb)

Liquid Measures

30ml	1 fluid oz
60ml	2 fluid oz
100ml	3 fluid oz
125ml	4 fluid oz
150ml	5 fluid oz (¼ pint)
190ml	6 fluid oz
250ml	8 fluid oz
300ml	10 fluid oz (½ pint)
500ml	16 fluid oz
600ml	20 fluid oz (1 pint)
1 litre	1¾ pints

INDEX

ABOUT THE AUTHORS

Ita Buttrose AO, OBE, Australian of the Year 2013
Ita Buttrose has been the Patron of the Macular Disease Foundation Australia since 2005. With members of her family affected by macular degeneration, Ita is keenly aware of the growing incidence and impact of the disease and is a passionate spokesperson for the Foundation. Her commitment to the cause, along with her enormous public profile and popularity, has been an invaluable contribution to the work of the Foundation and has helped elevate the profile of the disease in Australia. She has had a long involvement in many community health issues including breast and prostate cancer, HIV/AIDS, arthritis and Alzheimer's disease. She was made an Officer of the Order of Australia (AO) in 1988, for service to the community, particularly in the field of medical education and health care.

Ita has been a driving force in the development of this cookbook and donated her professional skills and time as editor. The Foundation extends its sincere gratitude for Ita's work and dedication.

Vanessa Jones is a talented chef who has worked at some of Australia's top restaurants and clubs. Most recently, as Executive Chef at the Union, University & Schools Club of Sydney, she was responsible for the running of the Club's dining and bar areas and for the serving of more than 1000 meals a week to its members and guests. Prior to that Vanessa was Executive Chef at Parliament House, Sydney. She now works as a private chef in the Southern Highlands of New South Wales where she now lives..

Born in 1979 at Wollongong on the South Coast of New South Wales, Vanessa trained at Wollongong TAFE and subsequently worked in a variety of leading kitchens including Hayman Island in Queensland, the Bathers' Pavilion at Sydney's Balmoral, and Milton Park Country House Hotel, Bowral. Vanessa was the former food writer and stylist for *Highlife*, one of the Southern Highlands' most popular magazines.

Eating for Eye Health is her first cookbook.

MACULAR DISEASE FOUNDATION AUSTRALIA

The Macular Disease Foundation Australia is a not-for-profit organisation meeting the needs of the macular disease community across Australia. Its mission is to reduce the incidence and impact of macular disease in Australia.

For more information or for a free comprehensive information kit, contact the Foundation:

Helpline: 1800 111 709

Email: info@mdfoundation.com.au

Website: www.mdfoundation.com.au

Level 9, 447 Kent Street Sydney NSW 2000

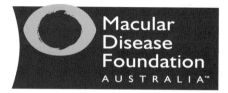

Our focus is your vision

UK £9.99

US $16.99